Praise for *A Nurse's S*
Writing Your Disser

"Finally, there is a clear, step-by-step guide for students—and faculty—on writing capstone papers and dissertations. From the first chapter on how to use this book to the practical review of basic (but sorely needed) writing skills at the end, Roush coaches readers through the scholarly writing process in an engaging, conversational style. I hope this book finds its way into the hands of anyone seeking to write a scholarly paper. It's certainly a resource I will be recommending."

–Maureen Shawn Kennedy, MA, RN, FAAN
Editor in Chief, *American Journal of Nursing*

"Roush's work has taken the mystery and confusion out of the often dreaded and frequently feared experience of writing a dissertation. In a clear, reader-friendly, engaging, and thorough manner, she has laid out an extremely helpful guide for those whose academic journey requires completion of this last step toward the prize. "

–Donna Sabella, PhD, MEd, MSN, CRNP-BC
Director of Global Studies
Drexel University College of Nursing and Health Professions

"Drawing on years of experience as editorial director and clinical managing editor, Roush provides a practical guide to the often overwhelming process of putting ideas succinctly on paper. With the help of many detailed examples, the author shows how each step can be confronted and completed efficiently in good time."

–Wendy C. Budin, PhD, RN-BC, FAAN
Director of Nursing Research, NYU Langone Medical Center
Adjunct Professor, New York University College of Nursing
Research Professor of Nursing, NYU School of Medicine

"The next generation of nurses to set off on that long, lonely quest of the finished dissertation or capstone will surely declare Karen Roush's new guidebook indispensable. Her voice is clear, straightforward, and unflappable. No doubt her readers will embrace this book—first page to last—as the trusted companion that saw them through."

–Madeleine Mysko, MA, RN
Contributing Editor, *American Journal of Nursing*

"A Nurse's Step-By-Step Guide to Writing Your Dissertation or Capstone gives practical guidance in a voice that seems at once trustworthy and wise. That's because Roush knows writing from every angle: as an editor, a nursing professor, and a writer of works both scholarly and creative. This book will prove itself essential for any nurse pursuing the PhD or DNP."

–Joy Jacobson, MFA
Adjunct Faculty, Hunter–Bellevue School of Nursing
Poet-in-Residence, Center for Health, Media, and Policy, Hunter College

"This book is a must-read for all doctoral students as they embark on their independent project as the last requirement for their degree. This is a well-written primer of practical advice on how to organize, stay focused, and most importantly, complete the project. This is the sage advice a student will rarely receive in the classroom or from faculty. I highly recommend this key resource to all doctoral students and their faculties."

–Jane Barnsteiner, PhD, RN, FAAN
Emeritus Professor, School of Nursing
University of Pennsylvania

"A Nurse's Step-by-Step Guide to Writing Your Dissertation or Capstone, is a "must-have" for all PhD and DNP scholars. The checklists, tips, examples, and resource lists are invaluable tools for success!"

–Darlene J. Curley, MS, RN, FAAN
Executive Director, Jonas Center for Nursing and Veterans Healthcare

"Roush has triumphed in her quest as writing mentor, as she has simplified and organized the process for the most daunting of research projects. This guide concisely outlines all elements of chapters, integrates crucial tips for formatting and preventing common errors, and most notably, eliminates the mystery of the construction of a dissertation, often the greatest obstacle to writing progress. *A Nurse's Step-By-Step Guide to Writing Your Dissertation or Capstone* should be required text for doctoral nursing students."

–Donna Rolin, PhD, APRN, PMHCNS-BC
Assistant Professor, Director of
Psychiatric Nurse Practitioner Graduate Program
University of Texas at Austin, School of Nursing

A NURSE'S STEP-BY-STEP GUIDE TO
WRITING YOUR DISSERTATION OR CAPSTONE

KAREN ROUSH, PhD, APN

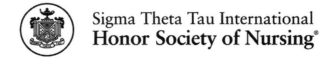

Sigma Theta Tau International
Honor Society of Nursing®

The Honor Society of Nursing, Sigma Theta Tau International (STTI) is a nonprofit organization found-ed in 1922 whose mission is to support the learning, knowledge, and professional development of nurses committed to making a difference in health worldwide. Members include practicing nurses, instructors, researchers, policymakers, entrepreneurs and others. STTI's 494 chapters are located at 676 institutions of higher education throughout Australia, Botswana, Brazil, Canada, Colombia, Ghana, Hong Kong, Japan, Kenya, Malawi, Mexico, the Netherlands, Pakistan, Portugal, Singapore, South Africa, South Korea, Swaziland, Sweden, Taiwan, Tanzania, United Kingdom, United States, and Wales. More information about STTI can be found online at www.nursingsociety.org.

Sigma Theta Tau International
550 West North Street
Indianapolis, IN, USA 46202

To order additional books, buy in bulk, or order for corporate use, contact Nursing Knowledge International at 888.NKI.4YOU (888.654.4968/US and Canada) or +1.317.634.8171 (outside US and Canada).

To request a review copy for course adoption, e-mail solutions@nursingknowledge.org or call 888.NKI.4YOU (888.654.4968/US and Canada) or +1.317.634.8171 (outside US and Canada).

To request author information, or for speaker or other media requests, contact Marketing, Honor Society of Nursing, Sigma Theta Tau International at 888.634.7575 (US and Canada) or +1.317.634.8171 (outside US and Canada).

ISBN: 9781940446080
EPUB ISBN: 9781940446097
PDF ISBN: 9781940446103
MOBI ISBN: 9781940446110

Library of Congress Cataloging-in-Publication Data

Roush, Karen, author.
  A nurse's step-by-step guide to writing your dissertation or capstone / Karen Roush.
    p. ; cm.
  Includes bibliographical references.
  ISBN 978-1-940446-08-0 (print : alk. paper) -- ISBN 978-1-940446-09-7 (EPUB) -- ISBN 978-1-940446-10-3 (PDF) -- ISBN 978-1-940446-11-0 (Mobi)
  I. Sigma Theta Tau International, issuing body. II. Title.
  [DNLM: 1. Education, Nursing--methods. 2. Writing. 3. Dissertations, Academic as Topic. WY 18]
  RT73
  610.73071'1--dc23
                        2015003590

Second Printing, 2016

Publisher: Dustin Sullivan
Acquisitions Editor: Emily Hatch
Editorial Coordinator: Paula Jeffers
Cover Designer: Rebecca Batchelor
Interior Design/Page Layout: Rebecca Batchelor

Principal Book Editor: Carla Hall
Development and Project Editor: Kevin Kent
Copy Editor: Keith Cline
Proofreader: Erin Geile
Indexer: Jane Palmer

Dedication

This book is dedicated to the NYU College of Nursing alumni out there who made the PhD journey with me. Our unshakeable belief in each other carried us through.

About the Author

Karen Roush, PhD, APN, is assistant professor of nursing at Lehman College in the Bronx, New York. She received her PhD in Nursing Research and Theory Development from the College of Nursing at New York University. She started her nursing education with an associate degree in nursing from Adirondack Community College in 1982, went on for her BSN at Russell Sage College, and then earned a master's degree at Columbia University in 1996, where she specialized as a family nurse practitioner.

Roush served for many years as editorial director and clinical managing editor for the *American Journal of Nursing (AJN)* and continues her affiliation with the journal as an editorial consultant. In addition, she is the founder of The Scholar's Voice, which works to strengthen the voice of nursing through writing mentorship for nurses. Widely published, she has authored multiple consumer healthcare books, numerous nursing articles in peer-reviewed journals, essays, and poetry. She is a regular blogger for *AJN*'s Off the Charts, and she advocates against gender-based violence by writing and speaking on the topic.

Roush received the award for Outstanding Doctoral Graduate at NYU College of Nursing in 2014 and the Fred Schmidt Award for Humanitarian Focused Research in 2011. She has traveled to Rwanda, Uganda, and India as a nursing volunteer and taught nursing students in Ghana. In addition, she was a visiting scholar in the Department of Human Resources for Health at the World Health Organization in Geneva, Switzerland.

Table of Contents

3   Writing Your Methodology Chapter 37

Preliminaries (AKA *Introduction to the Book*)

What Is This Book, Anyway?

This is a book about *writing* your dissertation or capstone. It is intentionally small because the last thing a doctoral candidate needs is another doorstop-sized book to buy, read, and lug around. This is a step-by-step guide to help you write your dissertation or capstone. It will not help you design or conduct research, but it will help you plan, document, organize, and write your dissertation or capstone.

What Will You Get From This Book?

Before I talk about what you'll get from this book, I want to talk about two essential things you need to successfully complete a dissertation or capstone that you won't get from this or any book: **perseverance** and a **community**.

Of all the characteristics you need to get through doctoral studies, the foremost is *perseverance*. Early in my studies, a student preparing for his final defense gave me the best piece of advice I ever got: "Just keep going; it's all about perseverance." That advice echoed reassuringly for me many, many times through the years. Because there will be days you will wonder if it's worth it, if you'll ever get there, if you'll ever hear that coveted title—Doctor—attached to *your* name. You will, if you persevere. You're smart enough, you already have a lot of the knowledge you need, and what you don't have you'll learn along the way. What really separates the perpetual ABDs (*all but dissertation*, three of the most frustrating words known to doctoral students) from the doctors is **perseverance.**

The other essential thing you won't get from this book is *a community of fellow students*. Hang on to each other; confer, curse, and cry together. No one else will understand what you are going through; people outside the experience have no concept of the exhilarating but often painful process of reimagining your worldview, of reconfiguring your brain. At times, it is so intense that you swear you can feel your synapses breaking and reconnecting in new and different ways.

So, when it all seems like too much, and when you hit those unexpected roadblocks and delays—and you will (more revisions than you anticipated, difficulty recruiting, conflicting advice from committee members)—gather your community around you and persevere. You *will* get there.

Okay, now on to what you will you get from this book.

This book takes you step by step through writing your dissertation or capstone, with chapters that correspond exactly with the chapters of a dissertation or capstone. There's no fluff here. No attempt to make the book look bigger to attract attention. All I intend to do is to help you successfully write your dissertation or capstone, and I've tried to do so in a succinct and logical way, with only the occasional interruption for important notes and tips gleaned the hard way.

HOW TO USE THIS BOOK

To get the most out of this book, you want to follow these three steps:

1. Do a quick read-through of the book to get an overall picture of what lies ahead and to check that you have included all required items in your planning and design.

2. Before you begin writing, read Chapter 6 on the craft of writing.

3. Before you start working on a particular section of your paper, carefully read the chapter in this book that applies to it.

Getting Started

Important Note: *Start your writing with Chapter Two (Literature Review), not Chapter One (Introduction).* That's because before you start writing, you need to know the literature inside out so that you thoroughly understand your topic, where your work fits in the context of prior research, and what relevant interventions have been tried. All of that comes from undertaking and writing the literature review. The introduction and background section is really a short synopsis of your literature review; so after you've completed Chapter Two, your literature review, you'll have everything you need to go back and write Chapter One, the introduction.

As mentioned previously, this book is not about how to design and conduct research or a quality-improvement project. However, you cannot produce a well-written dissertation or capstone if gaps exist in your thinking or planning, and using this book can help reveal them. When you do a first read-through of the book, note what is required to be included in each section. Make sure that you have included all of these elements when planning and designing your study or project.

The Purpose

Nothing is more important than your purpose statement; it is the whole reason for the dissertation or project. *Before doing anything, make sure that you have a clear, concise purpose statement.* Everything else flows from that.

Defining your purpose is a process that you cannot do quickly or in isolation. It is refined over time with the help of your mentors and committee members, through class discussions, dialogue with colleagues and fellow students, and just plain hard thinking about it again and again. Along the way, you will have done a preliminary literature review to get an idea of the state of the knowledge and the research gaps.

Once your purpose statement is done, you're ready to move on to the more comprehensive literature review and writing the dissertation or capstone project.

Once you have your purpose statement, print it in large font and prop it up or pin it on a bulletin board in front of you while you're working. *Everything* in your paper should be directly connected to that purpose statement. It's easy to go off on tangents as you get into the literature, so make sure that you can trace everything back to your study or project purpose statement.

Structure and Components of a Dissertation/Capstone

The overall structure of a dissertation and capstone is similar. A dissertation is the written report of an original research project, while a capstone is the written report of a quality-improvement or other project that translates evidence into practice. The structure of both is based on the recommendations of the International Committee of Medical Journal Editors (ICMJE) and the Standards for Quality Improvement Reporting Excellence (SQUIRE) guidelines.

ICMJE is used for reporting original research, and SQUIRE is used for reporting quality-improvement projects. But both follow the IMRAD structure: **i**ntroduction, **m**ethods, **r**esults, and **d**iscussion. A dissertation/capstone adds an additional section: an in-depth, comprehensive literature review.

Requirements will vary among different programs, so confirm your program's guidelines.

Dissertation Template

The dissertation is structured as five distinct chapters corresponding to IMRAD, with the literature review added as the second chapter. This template is fairly standard regardless of discipline or school. However, programs often have different specific requirements within that structure. So before beginning, carefully review your program's specific requirements. For the most part, your dissertation template will follow the outline discussed in this section.

Chapter One: Introduction

The introduction introduces the topic, provides some background information, explains why the topic is important, briefly describes what is known about the topic, states what we need to know, and concludes with the purpose of the dissertation research.

Chapter Two: Literature Review

The literature review (sometimes called a literature survey) gives an in-depth analysis of what is known about the topic through a review of the existing literature. It presents and summarizes the current knowledge on the topic and relevant concepts. It identifies gaps in knowledge and concludes with identification of the knowledge gap, how your dissertation research will address that gap (your purpose), research questions, and any hypotheses.

Chapter Three: Methodology

The methodology chapter describes in detail the study methods, including the theoretical frameworks, sampling, setting, ethical approvals, how the data will be collected, instruments that will be used for data collection, and how data analysis will be conducted.

Chapter Four: Results

The results chapter presents the findings. It includes the final sample size and demographics. Tables and figures are often used to report data.

Chapter Five: Discussion

The discussion chapter interprets the findings and compares them to findings in prior research on the topic. It also includes limitations and implications for practice and future research. The discussion chapter may also include a short conclusion that highlights the key points and wraps up.

Capstone Template

The capstone template is similar to that of the dissertation, but whereas the structure of a dissertation is usually standard among different schools and programs, the structure of the capstone varies somewhat. The IMRAD structure is still the foundation, and all the components of SQUIRE guidelines are still there, but where they are placed and what they are called can vary. Some structure the capstone into sections without distinct chapters. Others may use chapters, but what goes where may vary. For example, the literature review may be included as part of Chapter One, and Chapter Two describes the project (methods). The evaluation (analysis) may be separated from methods in its own chapter, as well. Outcomes (results) and implications (discussion) are always going to follow at the end of the paper, although there may be different specific requirements within them.

This book follows a structure that closely aligns to IMRAD and the SQUIRE guidelines and is very similar to the dissertation structure. When it differs, the text alerts you to that fact, and specific guidelines for capstones are provided where appropriate. The capstone template will follow the outline discussed in this section.

Chapter One: Introduction and Background

This chapter introduces the topic and explains why it is important. It also gives background information on the *local problem* (what is happening in your specific setting that requires improvement). It usually includes a problem statement section that may include the purpose of your project, a PICOT question, and objectives and aims.

Chapter Two: Literature Review

The literature review provides an in-depth analysis of what is known about the topic. It presents and summarizes the current knowledge on the topic and relevant concepts. It looks closely at the interventions related to your project that have been used and tested in the past. It also identifies gaps in knowledge. It concludes with a summary that leads to the purpose of your project. The theoretical framework is usually discussed in this chapter.

Chapter Three: Methods

This chapter describes the project. It includes the setting, people involved in the project, sample, ethical approvals, resources needed, outcomes, and how the project will be evaluated, including instruments. It also includes a timeline and budget.

Chapter Four: Results

The results chapter presents the outcomes of the project, usually organized by objective. It includes facilitators and barriers encountered during implementation. Tables and figures are often used to report data.

Chapter Five: Discussion

This chapter discusses the results of the project and the real-world experience of carrying out the project. It makes recommendations for the ongoing implementation of the project in your setting and for application of the project in other settings. It also includes limitations and unforeseen outcomes, both positive and negative. The discussion chapter may also include a short conclusion that highlights the key points and wraps up.

Tenses in a Dissertation/Capstone: Past, Present, or Future?

What tense you should be writing in can get confusing in dissertation and capstone papers. When you begin, you are writing a proposal for something you are going to do in the future. Once you complete the study or project, you are writing about something you did in the past. And then there are the parts of your dissertation or capstone where the tense isn't affected by whether you have done the study or project yet. Here are guidelines to follow:

- **Introduction:** Present tense for background unless you are talking about what an earlier study found. Then it is past tense. Future tense for what you propose to do when writing the proposal and past tense for what you did in the final dissertation/capstone paper.

- **Literature review:** Past tense for review of the literature. Present tense for research gaps. Future tense for how you are going to address it in the proposal, and past tense for how you addressed it in the final dissertation/capstone paper.

- **Methodology:** Future tense for proposal. Past tense for final dissertation/capstone paper.

- **Results:** Past tense.

- **Discussion:** What was in the literature and what your results were are in past tense. Implications for practice and research are in present and future tense.

When you've finished the research study or project and are writing your dissertation, remember to go back through the entire paper and change the tense from future to past where appropriate. You will need to do this primarily in the sections on methodology, data analysis, and outcomes, but also in parts of your introduction and literature review in which you talked about what you were planning to do.

General Tips and Recommendations

Following are some tips that can make the going a little smoother. Some are general for any writing you do, while others are specific to the dissertation/capstone journey. Taking some time upfront to prepare yourself to write, organizing your work and workspace, and using the resources available to you will alleviate some of the inevitable stress and frustrations ahead.

Read

Ask your committee members to recommend examples of well-written dissertations or capstones written by former students. You can find full-text dissertations and capstones online in the Dissertation Abstracts database (ProQuest), which is part of many colleges' digital database collections. Read through a few to get an idea of the structure, flow, depth of information, language, and length overall and of various sections.

Also read research and quality-improvement project reports in the biomedical literature. The more you are exposed to the language and the flow you find in those reports, the more natural they will be for you.

Befriend Your Research Librarian

Use your research librarian. Research librarians can help you greatly. They are experts in searching the literature and can help you set up a search strategy, find articles, and organize the results.

Use a Bibliographic Software Program

Bibliographic software programs are one of the greatest inventions when it comes to writing scholarly papers—especially long, complex ones like dissertations and capstones. With one of these programs, such as RefWorks or EndNote, you can save articles, organize your articles into folders, and—best of all—create reference lists in whatever format you need. You can usually sign up for an account through your school's library page; most schools provide student access for free. Don't be put off because you think you'll have to learn a complicated software program. The programs do have a variety of advanced features, but even used at their most basic level—saving articles and putting them in folders, formatting reference lists—they will save you countless hours of work.

- Check with your school's library for courses on using the programs or make an appointment with the librarian for a lesson. An hour or two spent learning a program now will pay off big later.

- As you do your literature review, throw into your account *every article you come across that relates to your topic.* Even if you don't think you will use it, you might. On many occasions, you will remember reading an article about something that would be helpful, and you will spend far too much time searching for it, often to never find it again (unless you follow the advice given here).

- Bibliographic programs aren't flawless. *So, always carefully check your reference list for errors.* Most of these are mistakes with capitalization; the programs do not always recognize proper nouns.

Get to Know Word

Most students have a basic proficiency with Microsoft's Word. Unless you're a professional writer, however, you're probably not nearly as proficient as you could be. Here again, taking a few hours in the beginning can save you a significant amount of time (and keystrokes) down the road. Instead of spending an hour trying to figure out how to go from portrait to landscape and back again for that figure or table, it's done in a minute. Check your college library for courses and sign up for one. When you are writing hundreds of pages (yes, with revisions you will be writing hundreds of pages before you're done), every keystroke saved makes a difference in time and frustration.

Get on the Cloud

Set up an account with one of the many cloud file-hosting programs, such as Google Docs or Dropbox. After you do, you can access your work anywhere there's a computer and an Internet connection. When you finish each work session, upload your latest version to the program. These services also provide other advantages; for example, you can share your work with other people, such as your committee members or colleagues, and you have the safety of file backup. If your computer crashes, the files are out there in cyberland waiting for you.

Designate a Dedicated Workspace

You want a place where you can have your work ready and waiting for you so that you can dive right in. You'll be creating all kinds of piles—types of articles, notes for different chapters, reference books—and you don't want to have to pick them all up and put them away and then take them all out and reorganize them again for each work session.

Also, you want a place where your mind and body know exactly what is expected of them when you are there—just as putting on running clothes and sneakers prepares you for running and putting on scrubs prepares you to work.

Make the Time

You will never "find" time to write. It's not lost somewhere out there; it just doesn't exist. So you need to make it. And once you do, prioritize it. Nothing interferes with the time you have reserved for writing. Period. Not laundry, not that junk drawer you've been meaning to clean out for the past 6 months, not the really fascinating list of ingredients on the back of the cereal box.

And especially not the endless distractions to be found on the Internet. Banish YouTube from your life. Declare a moratorium on FreeCell and the hundred other solitaire variations calling to you.

You need to really focus on your work during the time you make for it. A dissertation or capstone is a creative process that requires a level of critical thinking that can only be achieved with uninterrupted, focused attention. When your mind starts wandering, take 15 minutes to go for a walk or run, meditate, or take a nap; then go back to work with *100%* concentration.

Gather

Keep a dissertation/capstone notebook. Write down ideas, quotes, questions, names of people you come across who are working in your field, programs related to what you are doing—anything that may be useful, even if indirectly. Developing a dissertation or capstone is an ongoing iterative process; you will find yourself constantly thinking about it, breaking it down, adding and deleting, and reconfiguring. Have a place to save it all, and come back to things when needed.

Don't Start at the Beginning

If you have ever attended a writing workshop or read a book on the writing process, you have probably heard this already. Every writer dreads the blank page, and starting with what feels easiest or is uppermost in your mind can help overcome that. As noted previously in this chapter, when writing a dissertation or capstone, it's preferable not to start at the beginning, because everything you need for the introduction is in the literature review. But you can also start writing part of the methods section or the theoretical framework or any other area you feel ready to put down on paper.

Save Every Copy Every Time

Each time you work on your paper, save it as a new version. As you proceed there will be times you decide that an earlier draft of something you wrote is actually better, or something you decided to delete actually belongs in the paper after all. When you save your changes as separate versions, you will be able to go back and pull out whatever you need. If you are doing a lot of work at one sitting with many changes, then you may even consider saving multiple versions during that work period. To save your work as a different version, use the Save As command and change the name slightly each time. You can go in alphabetical order and assign a letter to each version, for example you can save versions as Lit_Review_a, Lit_Review_b, Lit_Review_c, and so forth. Or you can use the date for each version; Capstone_032815, Capstone_033015, and if there are multiple versions in one day, add a letter to each version: Capstone_032815a, Capstone_032814b.

Organize Your Work

Create folders on your computer for all your drafts. Have a folder for each chapter, for the drafts of the complete proposal (Chapters One through Three), and one for the drafts of the final dissertation or capstone (Chapters One through Five). If you print out hard copies of articles included in the literature review, jot notes on the first page that will tell you at a glance what key points that article is contributing to the review, and organize the articles in piles by variable, concept, or topic. Articles within each pile can be organized in alphabetical order by author. That way you can quickly find a specific article or flip through the pile and look at the notes you made to find an article with the information you need. For example, in my dissertation on intimate partner violence in the rural setting, I had piles labeled incidence/prevalence, physical consequences, mental health consequences, economic costs, isolation, leaving, and risk factors, among others.

Follow Requirements for Your Program

This book presents the most common structures and requirements for a dissertation or capstone project. Your program may have specific requirements that differ from what is covered here. As noted previously, make sure that you follow your program's specific requirements.

In addition, *always follow the directions of your chairperson and other committee members*. If they insist on a particular format or writing style, do it their way. For example, many academicians still insist that the first-person point of view should not be used in scholarly papers. If your committee members are among them, don't use the first person.

Remember, the best dissertation is a done dissertation! And your committee will determine when that is the case. So, cede to their directives when necessary.

Academic Integrity

Please, please, please pay careful attention to issues of academic integrity! Do not be complacent or think this doesn't apply to you. Plagiarism is an ongoing problem in academia. Some of it is intentional appropriation of another's work, usually when copying material from a source. But sometimes it is the result of a lack of understanding of what constitutes plagiarism.

We all know that taking something word-for-word from a published or nonpublished source is plagiarism. However, that is only one type of plagiarism. Other types you have to watch out for are the use of someone else's ideas without giving proper attribution or following too close to the source, such as when paraphrasing.

Make sure you always give credit where credit is due. If you are using an argument presented elsewhere, or building on another's ideas, you must give them credit.

Considering the ideas about repressed grief put forth by Smith (1998)...

As Smith (1998) argued...

I agree with Smith (1998), who posited that...

Be careful with paraphrasing. It is not good enough to just change the wording if the material presented is essentially the same as the original. If it is not your synthesis or interpretation of information, then you should be giving attribution to the original source.

With the ability to use cut and paste tools, it is very easy to accidentally include fragments pasted from other documents in your own work. **Never cut and paste information from an article or other source directly into your Word document,** even with the intention of rewriting. I have heard from many students and authors who have been caught plagiarizing that they did this and then either used the wrong draft or, for one reason or another, inadvertently overlooked rewriting the pasted material in their own words.

Do not risk your degree or your academic future—watch out for plagiarism.

Finally...

Use the following checklist to set yourself up to succeed.

Checklist for Success

Have I...

- ❑ Set up my writing space?

- ❑ Scheduled dedicated writing times?

- ❑ Read sample dissertation or capstone projects?

- ❑ Reviewed my program's dissertation or capstone requirements and guidelines?

- ❑ Set up Google Docs, Dropbox, or a similar cloud account?

- ❑ Written a clear, focused purpose statement?

- ❑ Made an appointment with a research librarian?

- ❑ Reviewed ICMJE and SQUIRE guidelines?

- ❑ Set up a bibliographic software account?

You've worked so hard to get to this point. Don't let writer's block or an unorganized approach slow you down toward your goal to get it done! This book will help you in many ways, so keep it handy at all times. Whenever you get stuck or find yourself blocked, remember those key elements I mentioned at the beginning of this introduction: **perseverance** and **community**.

Now, go forward and get it done!

–Karen Roush

1

WRITING YOUR INTRODUCTION

ELEMENTS OF YOUR INTRODUCTION

1. Provides some background information so that readers understand the issue

2. Explains why the issue is important

3. Describes what is known about the issue

4. States what we need to find out or what action needs to be taken and why

5. Presents how you plan to do that (your study/project)

There's a good reason you chose your dissertation or capstone topic. Maybe an experience in your personal life left you determined to make things better for others experiencing the same thing. Or perhaps you've witnessed too many patients having poor outcomes after a certain procedure, and you want to figure out a way to change that. Perhaps you chose in response to lack of knowledge or poor attitudes about a particular condition that causes unnecessary suffering for those who experience it. Or you've noticed a systems issue that is creating increased work stress for fellow nurses.

Whatever it is, something made you sit up and pay attention. The introduction is your opportunity to make the reader do the same. In this part of the dissertation, you tell the reader *why* you care about this topic, and even more important, why they should care too.

In dissertation/capstone speak, we call this *establishing significance*. In plain English, we're saying, "Hey, listen up! This is important, and here's why."

Of course, you can't expect the reader to just take your word for it. You need to first give them information so that they understand the problem, and you need to back up that information with evidence. After you do that, you can ask them to consider your idea for what we need to do next, whether that is gathering more information or trying out a solution.

You've Already Started

Good news: You've already done most of the work for this chapter! Most of the introduction is going to come from all the information you gathered when you did your literature review. What you want to do is summarize the literature review. As you do so, include enough information to familiarize readers with your topic and convince them of its importance without extensive details or in-depth review of individual studies.

Create an Outline

You can begin by developing an outline based on the required elements. To do so, first answer each of the following questions (which correlate with required elements one through four listed at the beginning of this chapter) with one or two sentences:

1. What is happening?

2. Why should we care?

3. What do we know now?

4. What do we need to find out and why?

If you have a hard time keeping your answers to one or two sentences, you might need to refine your study/project to focus it more. Get rid of any noise, all that extraneous information that is not really bringing value to the paper. It's the old *need to know vs. nice to know*. In a dissertation/capstone, we only want the *need to know* stuff. If information isn't adding value to the paper, it's distracting from it and may even confuse the reader. In photography, we call this narrowing the f-stop (focusing in on the intended subject and letting everything else blur out so that the viewer's eye goes right to what's important).

KEEP IT OR DELETE IT?

Remember: Stay focused on your purpose statement. Keep it in sight—prop it up next to your computer or tape it to the wall in front of you, Go back to it whenever you start adding information to the paper and ask yourself these two questions:

1. Is this information directly related to my purpose statement?

2. Does it add to the reader's understanding of the problem, topic, or concept?

If the answer to either one of these is no, delete it. Be ruthless with yourself. Conciseness means clarity—make that your mantra.

After you have answered the questions, read your answers in order. Each answer should connect with what comes before and all of them should lead you straight to a logical *therefore* statement.

> *Therefore, I am going to conduct a study to…*

> *Therefore, we designed a quality-improvement project to…*

If the answers don't lead directly to the *therefore* statement, what is missing? Where does the connection get lost? If you haven't gotten the reader to care, then it doesn't matter what you know and what you want to do. Or maybe now the reader cares but wonders why you need to do this particular study at this particular time, because it doesn't seem to be the next logical thing to do based on what's already been done.

Here is an example of what the answers to these questions might be for the dissertation proposal on IPV in the rural setting:

1. What is happening?

   Intimate partner violence (IPV) is a pervasive health and social problem in the United States. One out of three women experiences IPV in her lifetime.

2. Why should we care?

   It causes tremendous physical and emotional suffering and even death. It's costly to individual women and society.

3. What do we know now?

   Women in the rural setting who experience IPV face unique challenges. Current support and resources are inadequate and ineffective.

4. What do we need to find out and why?

There is little research on the lived experience of IPV for women in the rural setting. We need to understand this so we can develop effective services and provide appropriate resources and support.

Therefore, I propose a qualitative descriptive study of the lived experience of women who experience intimate partner violence in the rural setting.

After you've answered the questions satisfactorily, have someone unfamiliar with the topic area take a look at it. Does that person agree that the *therefore* statement makes perfect sense? If not, back to the drawing board. If they do, *brava*, you're on your way.

 You need to consider these questions and review your answers carefully. They represent the very basis for your study.

How you proceed at this point depends on your own writing work style. Some people prefer to work from a detailed outline. If you do, you can now begin to fill in your answers with more particulars. If you are not an outline type of worker, you can move on to writing the introduction, as described later in this chapter.

Filling In the Outline

Under each question, list the different pieces of information that you need to add. Depending on your topic and purpose, your outline should include some or all of the following information:

1. What is happening?
   a. condition, problem, issue
      i. definition or brief description
      ii. population affected

   b. epidemiology

      i. how many

      ii. how often

      iii. where (e.g., United States, globally, developing countries, hospital or community)

      iv. mortality rates

   c. local problem (for quality-improvement project)

   d. associated concepts necessary to understanding of problem or approach

2. Why should we care?

   a. pain and suffering it causes

   b. mortality

   c. costs

      i. individual

      ii. organization/institution

      iii. society

   d. increasing or worsening?

   e. consequences/impact of local problem

3. What do we know now?

   a. recent research

   b. current treatments or interventions

      i. outcomes

      ii. limitations

4. What do we need to find out and why?

   a. questions that still need to be answered

   b. interventions to be trialed

    c. specific population

    d. benefits to be gained

        i. better patient outcomes

       ii. more effective interventions

      iii. improved services

      iv. workforce issues

       v. improved systems

Writing the Introduction

When you start writing this part of your dissertation, remember that each section is an *introduction* to the material included. So, do not get too detailed. The important thing is that you adequately and succinctly cover all these areas. In your literature review (Chapter Two), you critically review prior research and cover the individual studies in depth. In the introduction, in contrast, you present what is known with appropriate citations of the evidence but do not get into detailed information about that evidence.

In addition, you will notice some overlap among the four questions. Do not try to adhere to a structure that rigidly partitions answers to each question. For example, when you talk about prevalence in answer to the "What is happening?" question, you are beginning to make a case for significance.

What Is Happening?

The first paragraph introduces your topic and makes a brief statement about its significance. Within the first two sentences, the reader should know what the topic is. Don't take the reader on a roundabout trip to your topic. If your topic is stress incontinence in older women, start with a statement about stress incontinence. Do not start by talking about the aging of the population and then explain how older people have more problems with incontinence and that there are different types of incontinence, one of which is stress incontinence. Try to get the topic in the first sentence. After we know you're talking about stress incontinence, you can go on to tell us that it is more common in older women and that its prevalence is increasing with the aging of the population.

Describe the population that is affected and provide statistics on the prevalence:

- How many people are affected, or how often does it happen?
- How big is this problem?
- What population is primarily affected?
- What are the mortality and morbidity rates?
- Is the problem increasing, or is its impact becoming greater?

Remember to write from the general to the specific. So your first paragraph will state the problem and its prevalence and make a general statement about its impact. Then succeeding paragraphs will provide more details that will add to the reader's understanding of the topic, its significance, and related concepts.

For a capstone project, make sure you get to the *specific* problem you are addressing early in the introduction. A common mistake people make is starting with general background information and not mentioning the problem until many paragraphs or even pages into the introduction.

For example, if your project is looking at the role of teamwork in improving patient safety in the operating room (OR), state that in the first paragraph. Don't go on for a paragraph or two talking about patient safety in general or the importance of teamwork in healthcare overall. You can include that information in your literature review, but in the introduction you want to make sure that your reader knows exactly what your topic is from the beginning. So, you could begin your introduction with a statement about patient safety and the high rate of medical errors, particularly in high-risk environments such as the operating room. Then continue with information specific to the OR, including teamwork.

In a capstone project, you also have to give the reader background information on the "local problem." What is happening in your specific setting that compels you to do this quality-improvement project? How do you know there is a problem? What is the population affected? What are the consequences of the problem?

Check with your committee chair about using the name of your facility or organization in your paper. Guidelines on this vary. If your program's guidelines recommend using the name, then also check with administration at your facility or organization for what their policy is regarding using the name in papers and publications.

Why Should We Care?

Now that the reader knows what you're going to be talking about, you need to convince them of its importance. You do this by talking about the number of those affected by it and its impact on society. If you haven't talked about prevalence, an important aspect of a problem's significance, you will want to discuss it here.

The impact on those it affects is the other important aspect of a problem's significance. Depending on your topic this may include any of the following:

- Physical and mental health effects
- Social implications

- Economic impact on the individual and society
- Contribution to healthcare costs
- Healthcare system implications
- Patient safety outcomes
- Impact on the nursing profession

Be careful how and where you talk about the economic costs of a problem. You don't want it to appear that you are prioritizing cost over people. If your purpose is related to a health systems problem, economic costs may be a primary factor. However, if it is related to a patient outcomes problem, cost may be one of the reasons we should care, but it should not be the primary one. This can be made clear in the wording and where in the text you place information. If it is a patient-related problem, talk about cost last and begin with a transitional phrase such as *in addition to* or *along with* [the impact on patient]....

> *In addition to the decrease in patient suffering and lower risk of death, improving our CLABSI rates will result in significant cost savings to the hospital.*

What Do We Know Now?

You will have included some of what we know now in answering the first two questions. In answering this question, though, you want to talk about what is known *in relation to the specific purpose of your study or project.* This will then lead the reader to what we need to find out, which is the knowledge or practice gap that your dissertation or capstone is trying to fill.

If your study or project is looking to better understand a problem or discover more information about the impact of a problem, then in this section you will describe current understanding or information. If you are doing an interventional study or quality-improvement project that looks at how to address a problem, you also need to describe what we currently know about what works or doesn't work (in other words, what's already been tried and how it worked out).

What Do We Need to Find Out and Why?

Now that you've established where we're at currently, it's time to let the reader know what the next step should be. This is where you introduce the knowledge or practice gap that you are going to address in your study or project. This will be a shorter version of what you discuss in the literature review, but the same format applies. Use a transitional sentence to move from what is known to what we need to find out, or from what is known about a problem to what you are proposing to do about the problem. Then tell the reader why the knowledge or project is necessary.

But remember, keep it brief. One or two sentences should cover it.

> *Though there is evidence from studies of disenfranchised grief to suggest that parents who experience the death of an estranged son or daughter may suffer complicated grief and receive less support than other bereaved parents, there is little research that explores this experience in this population. Understanding the lived experience of grief after the death of an estranged son or daughter is needed for us to develop effective counseling and support services for these parents.*

And finally, what you are going to do:

> *Therefore, I am going to conduct a qualitative phenomeno-logical study of the meaning of grief in parents following the death of an estranged son or daughter.*

If you've done your job well, the *therefore* statement is inevitable. The reader is already there thinking, well, of course now you have to do that! Everything that came before has led directly to it.

PAST, PRESENT, OR FUTURE?

When writing your dissertation/capstone proposal, the statement will be in the future tense. After conducting the study, you will go back and revise it to be in the past tense for your final paper.

> *Therefore, I propose a quasi-experimental study to examine the effect of simulation teamwork exercises on the perception of teamwork among interprofessional operating room staff.*

> *Therefore, I conducted a descriptive qualitative study exploring the lived experience of intimate partner violence in women living in the rural setting.*

Purpose Statements

Your *therefore* statement may be worded as a purpose statement (the *therefore* is implied). Either way, make sure to state it *clearly* and *concisely*.

PURPOSE STATEMENT EXAMPLES

The purpose of this quality-improvement project is to determine whether biweekly home visits to heart-failure patients post hospital discharge conducted by a nurse practitioner will decrease 30-day readmission rates.

The purpose of this study was to determine the IPV-related knowledge, attitudes, beliefs, and behaviors of nurse practitioners practicing in a rural outpatient clinic.

PICOT Statements

You may be directed to write a PICOT problem statement, particularly if you are doing quantitative research or a quality-improvement capstone project.

Population: Who is the focus of your study or project?

Intervention: What activity/behavior is being tested?

Comparison: What group are you comparing your population to?

Outcome: What are the outcomes you are examining?

Time: What is the duration of the intervention?

PICOT STATEMENT EXAMPLE

Patients with heart failure have high readmission rates. I propose implementing a discharge follow-up program that provides biweekly post-discharge home visits by nurse practitioners for 2 weeks following hospital discharge. I will compare 30-day readmission rates for patients during the 6 months prior to initiation of the program and for the 6 months after initiation of the program.

Population: Patients discharged from the hospital with a diagnosis of heart failure

Intervention: Biweekly home visits by nurse practitioners

Comparison: Patients discharged prior to implementation of the intervention to patients discharged after implementation

Outcome: 30-day readmission rates

Time: 2 weeks

Not all purpose statements or research questions can be formulated into a PICOT problem statement. If you are doing a qualitative study, you might not have an intervention, comparison, outcome, or time.

Your Plan (Methodology)

After you state your purpose, you need to briefly describe how you propose to accomplish it. If you are doing a research study, your purpose statement usually includes the methodological approach you plan to use (as shown in the preceding examples). You should then describe your design in one or two sentences. Are you going to use a survey? Conduct interviews? Do focus groups? What is the sampling frame? Duration of the project or study period?

> *Therefore, I propose a discharge follow-up program for heart-failure patients that provides biweekly home visits by nurse practitioners for 2 weeks following hospital discharge. I will compare 30-day readmission rates for patients during the 6 months prior to initiation of the program and for the 6 months after initiation of the program.*

Research Questions

Finally, you include your specific research question or questions. This is usually your purpose statement reformulated as a question but may also include additional questions that drill down into more specifics.

> *What is the lived experience of IPV for women in the context of the rural setting?*

> *What are the IPV-related knowledge, attitudes, beliefs, and behaviors of healthcare providers in the rural setting?*

> *Will biweekly home visits conducted by nurse practitioners for 2 weeks post hospital discharge reduce readmission rates for heart-failure patients?*

Does participation in simulation teamwork exercises improve the perception of teamwork among interprofessional operating room staff?

If you have specific hypotheses, you include those in this section as well.

Checking That You've Covered Your Purpose Statement

When you finish the introduction, go back and check that all aspects of your purpose or *therefore* statement have been covered. Break the purpose statement into questions and check that each question is answered, albeit briefly, in the introduction. Not knowing the answer to any of the questions reveals gaps in your thinking or in your review of the literature.

Nothing about your purpose statement should be arbitrary. You should be able to clearly see where it came from: What in the literature or your practice supports your decisions about variables, time duration, and outcome measures?

So, let's look at the example of the discharge follow-up program for heart failure patients.

Therefore, I propose a discharge follow-up program that provides biweekly home visits by nurse practitioners for 2 weeks following hospital discharge. I will compare 30-day readmission rates for patients during the 6 months prior to initiation of the program and for the 6 months after initiation of the program.

For this purpose statement, you would want to be able to answer the following questions:

- Why look at a discharge follow-up program for heart-failure patients?

- Why post-discharge home visits as the follow-up intervention?

- Why make the visits biweekly?

- Why by nurse practitioners (vs. other healthcare personnel)?

- Why 2 weeks duration following hospital discharge?

- Why 30-day readmission rates as the outcome measure?

Of course, you will only be able to answer all the questions if your literature review was comprehensive and complete. If you haven't answered all these questions in the introduction, go back to your literature review and see whether the answers are there. If not, you've got to get back into the literature and find them and revise your literature review to include that information before moving on.

If you can answer all the questions, then onward to Chapter Two!

Chapter Checkup

❏ Have I convinced the reader of the importance of the study or project?

❏ Have I included enough background information for readers to understand the problem or issue and its context?

❏ Does the information provided lead logically and inevitably to the purpose statement?

❏ Is all the information directly related to my purpose statement?

❏ Have I gotten feedback?

❏ Have I clearly identified the research gap?

❏ Have I included all the information needed to support all the components of my purpose statement?

WRITING YOUR LITERATURE REVIEW

ELEMENTS OF THE LITERATURE REVIEW

1. Overview of what the chapter covers

2. Definitions of variables and concepts

3. Theoretical framework

4. Review of the literature

5. Summary

6. Research gaps

7. Purpose statement

In Chapter Two, you give readers everything they need to know to understand what you are researching or what issue you are addressing and why. It provides context for your study or project, establishing significance for the topic and answering the question of why your study or project should be done. It does this through a comprehensive literature review. The purpose of the literature review is for you to critically analyze and synthesize all the available literature on your topic, in addition to the literature on important concepts related to what you are doing.

> Analysis and synthesis are the hallmark of scholarly writing. You need to sift through the research for what is relevant, critically appraise it to see whether you can use the findings with confidence, and pull it all together to create a new understanding in the context of your research question.
>
> Also, research is a building process. Each study builds on what came before. In a dissertation literature review, you show how your work is the logical next building block in that process.

Chapter One and Chapter Two of the proposal, the introduction and the literature review, are very similar. In Chapter One, you introduce the topic to your readers and convince them of its importance and of the necessity of your study or project. You will do the same here in the literature review, but whereas the introduction "introduces" the study or project and provides a brief summary of relevant literature, the literature review goes into much greater detail and provides an in-depth analysis of the literature. Both the introduction and the literature review chapters end with the purpose of your study or project. All the information and how it is organized should lead readers directly and logically to that purpose.

> Remember to check your school's guidelines for specifics on the required organization of the literature review.

Begin With an Overview and Definitions

You want to begin your literature review chapter with a one-paragraph (or short) overview of what the chapter includes, describing specific areas that you will cover.

OVERVIEW EXAMPLE

Chapter Two, "Literature Review," includes a description of the theoretical framework and a review of the literature on intimate partner violence (IPV) in general and in women who experience IPV in the rural setting specifically. This review is divided into the following sections: a) Epidemiology, b) IPV risk factors, c) Help-Seeking and Leaving Abusive Relationships, d) Physical and Mental Health Consequences, e) Economic Costs of IPV to Society and to Women Who Experience IPV, f) IPV in Women in the Rural Setting, and g) Interactions with the Healthcare System.

Before proceeding with the literature review, you must define all the variables (operational definitions) and concepts included in your study/project to ensure that everyone is working from the same definitions. You can begin the definitions with the phrase *"For the purposes of this study, [concept] is defined as…,"* or you can simply state the definition.

In some programs, you will be required to include a separate list of definitions in the introduction or literature review or as an appendix. Check your program's guidelines. Even if this is not a requirement, you might want to do so if your dissertation contains many technical terms or complex concepts that could be unknown to or misinterpreted by the reader.

TERM/CONCEPT DEFINITIONS EXAMPLE

For the purposes of this study, the CDC definition of IPV, "physical, sexual or psychological harm by a current or former partner or spouse," is used (CDC, p. 1).

An area is considered rural if it does not contain any core urbanized areas, defined as a "delineated urban cluster of at least 50,000 or a Census Bureau delineated urban cluster of at least 10,000 population" (Office of Management and Budget, 2010, p. 37249) (Roush, 2014).

Explaining Your Theoretical Framework

An explanation of the theoretical framework of your dissertation is usually included as part of the literature review chapter, although some programs might require you to include it as a separate section in the introduction or in the methodology chapter (Chapter Three). As part of this explanation, you need to describe what theoretical model you are using, including its origin and precepts. Explain how it applies to your study or project.

Include an illustration that shows the theoretical framework/model as it applies to your project. Insert the study variables or concepts into the appropriate areas of the model. For example, the theoretical model for the IPV study was Bronfenbrenner's ecological systems model. The figure with the concepts applied looks like Figure 2.1.

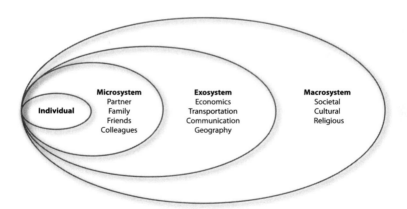

Figure 2.1   Theoretical model illustration example

Explaining Your Search Strategy

Most dissertations and capstones do not include the detailed search strategy in the literature review, but refer to your program's requirements to determine whether you need to describe yours in your paper. Regardless of whether the search strategy needs to be included, it is very important that you do your literature search in a systematic way to avoid bias. This way you won't "cherry pick" the studies that support your point of view or the preconceived ideas you have about your topic. As noted earlier, having the research librarian help you is the best way to ensure that you complete a comprehensive search of the literature.

A well-written search strategy is described in such a way that anyone replicating your search would come up with the same results. Read through a number of literature reviews and systematic reviews, and you will see that there is a certain formula for describing search strategies.

Elements of a well-reported search strategy include the following:

1. What topic you searched for

2. What databases you searched

3. Other sources searched, including gray literature

4. What keywords were used

5. What date delimitations were set and why

6. Number of studies found

7. Inclusion criteria that were applied and why

8. Number of studies remaining after inclusion criteria applied

9. Hand searching of bibliographies of remaining studies

10. Number of studies found with hand searching

11. Exclusion criteria that were applied and why

12. Number of studies remaining after exclusion criteria were applied

13. Any of these studies that were not included and why

14. Total number of studies included in review

15. General information on studies included (type, samples)

16. What of importance was *not* found

 If you had the help of a librarian, include that fact in the description of your search strategy with a statement such as *"Research librarian assisted in the search."*

You can see some of these elements numbered in the search strategy description that follows.

The literature review should include current research on your topic (published within the past 5 years), in addition to classic and seminal articles. You decide what dates to set as parameters when searching the literature (date delimitations). You must have a reason for choosing those dates; they are not arbitrary. For example, the dates might reflect when a policy change took effect, when a seminal study changed practice (such as the Women's Health Initiative studies did for use of postmenopausal hormone therapy), or when a new treatment became the standard of practice. If you decide to include a seminal or classic article that lies outside the date delimitations, just state that in the description of the search strategy.

SEARCH STRATEGY DESCRIPTION

I performed a literature search for all English-language studies on IPV in the rural setting (1). I searched Medline, Psychinfo, CINAHL, PubMed, and Google Scholar (2) for original research studies on IPV in the rural setting using the following keywords: "intimate partner violence," "domestic violence," "spousal abuse," and "battered women" combined with the keyword "rural" (4). Date delimitations were 1990 to the present, as sociocultural norms and IPV-related policies change over time (5). The search yielded 537 studies (6). After applying the inclusion criteria as outlined below, there were 76 studies remaining (8).

Inclusion criteria were original research studies or systematic reviews in peer-reviewed journals that examined IPV in adult women (18 years and older) in the rural setting in Western countries. Non-Western countries were not included because of differences in sociocultural norms that would influence the understanding and experience of IPV (7). Exclusion criteria were studies that had a narrow focus, such as smoking in rural pregnant women experiencing IPV; studies that were conducted in a rural setting but did not consider its implication, such as those that looked at instrument development, and studies with a narrow focus on specific populations in the rural area, such as migrant farm workers, where the findings were not generalizable to a broader rural population of women (11). In addition, studies of prevalence and incidence from prior to 2000 were excluded to include only more recent statistics (11).

After applying exclusion criteria, there were 36 studies remaining (12). Of these, 27 were quantitative, five were qualitative, one was ethnographic, and three were mixed methods studies (15).

If you include gray literature, you need to clearly identify it as such. Gray literature is information found outside of the usual bibliographic sources. This might include articles, technical reports, conference reports, reports from recognized organizations working in the topic area (such as NGOs), committee reports, white papers, or unpublished research reports.

Exclusion criteria are not the opposite of inclusion criteria. They are applied after inclusion criteria. So if a characteristic is not present in what you include, it should not be part of the exclusion criteria.

For example, if one of your inclusion criteria is women between the ages of 18 and 35, you will not have women younger than 18 or older than 35 as exclusion criteria because there won't be anyone younger than 18 or older than 35 to exclude.

As you do your literature search, save a PDF copy of each article to your computer and organize them into folders by topic. For example, for a capstone that addresses patient education in heart-failure patients, you might have folders for epidemiology, patient education, heart failure readmissions, self-management in heart failure, medication adherence, measurement of patient education outcomes, and so on. If you print articles, write a brief note in large print on the front page that clearly indicates what the article contributes. Then place them in piles by topic and clip an index card with the topic on the top article. (If you like working with hard copies, you'll find that the piles quickly become too large for actual folders.) If possible, clear space on the floor next to where you work and keep the piles spread out, or if there isn't enough room (or you have a small child or dog that will think the piles are great play material), then pile them in alphabetical order. The key is to make it quick and easy to find any article by topic when it's needed.

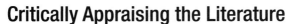

Critically Appraising the Literature

You must critically read each study that you include in the review of your literature. It is usually not necessary to grade the evidence or include an evidence table in your literature review (refer to your program's guidelines for specific instructions), but you should comment on the quality of the studies, when appropriate, in the review.

Along with critically analyzing individual studies, you need to analyze each study against the body of research. This is part of synthesizing the literature. If the results of one study conflict with multiple other studies, comment on this and consider possible explanations. If there are a number of weak studies on a phenomenon, but all had the same results, note that. As you synthesize the literature, note where the supporting evidence is weak or strong and any limitations that might have affected outcomes that are related to your study or project. Also note when results might or might not be applicable to your study setting or population.

CRITICAL APPRAISAL EXAMPLES

However, the project was conducted in a small rural hospital, and therefore its results might not be applicable to a large urban facility.

Though the project participants reported low satisfaction with the intervention, they also reported higher levels of chronic pain, and this might have affected the outcome.

However, these findings must be considered in the context of other studies, which consistently find that....

Numerous tools are available for appraising research reports (see the end of this chapter). These tools are also great for appraising your own work, as well. After completing the methodology chapter of the proposal, check its completeness and rigor using an appraisal tool that is appropriate for the type of study or project you are doing. You can do the same with the results and discussion chapters when you finish the study or project.

Synthesizing Your Research

Synthesis is the bigger picture that is created when information from individual studies is weaved together and presented in the context of your study/project. It's like constructing a jigsaw puzzle; all the studies are individual pieces, and you have to fit them together to create the bigger picture.

You want to organize your literature review around the variables, concepts, and factors involved in your study. The most common mistake people make is talking about each study individually without ever integrating the information from the studies together to create an understanding of or to make a statement about a variable, concept, or factor. If your literature review reads like a list of studies, talking about each study separately, one after the other, then you are not synthesizing.

A FEW WORDS ABOUT DIRECT QUOTES

Synthesis is your analysis and interpretation of the literature. As such there should be very few, if any, direct quotations used in your review. There are only a couple of good reasons to use a direct quotation in a literature review:

- The original is worded in an especially engaging or insightful way

- To rewrite would risk misinterpretation or loss of meaning

And remember, any time you use a direct quote you *must put it in quotation marks* and include a page number with the citation. Just citing the source is not enough; without quotation marks, it's considered plagiarism.

One approach to help you synthesize is to begin the section about a particular variable or concept with a general summary statement about that variable or concept and then follow with pertinent details from individual studies.

Synthesis is difficult. Everyone struggles with it in the beginning. Here is one technique to try:

- Make a list of the variables and concepts that are involved in your study/project. Write each one at the top of a separate piece of paper.

- Go through the studies you found and see what each said (relevant findings) about that particular aspect of the topic and write it down on the paper. Use charts, tables, and diagrams to organize what you found or to illustrate connections. (These are just for your use; they are not part of the paper.)

- Examine what you have on the page. What does all of that information tell us about that particular variable/concept? Write that up as a section of your literature review.

- Now, pull it all together and tell the reader—accurately, clearly, and directly—what the current knowledge is on your topic. Do not be afraid to make definitive statements when you can support them with evidence.

SYNTHESIZING EXAMPLE

The following example of synthesizing research is from an integrative review of the social implications of obstetric fistula, a devastating childbirth injury that occurs in developing countries. This paragraph describes the role that stigmatization plays in isolating the women studied:

There were consistent reports across all studies of stigmatization coming from the woman's own family, who may give her food and shelter but segregate her for eating and sleeping and not allow her to participate in household activities. Women in the Turan et al.[19] study reported that family members made them live separately due to their smell; Ojanuga[18] related how one woman's family mocked her; Muleta et al.[20] quoted a woman as saying, "My parents really disliked me for the stench coming from me; they made me sleep on a bare floor"; and the Women's Dignity Project and EngenderHealth study[16] related the case of a 20-year-old woman whose grandmother told her "Get lost, I am fed up. I can't put up with your smell!" Quantitative data from Murphy[15] indicate that like that of the husband's support, family's support diminishes over time; for the first hospital visit 27% of the women arrived alone and on subsequent visits 78% arrived alone (Roush, 2009).

Studies often disagree, and that is okay. Part of your job in the review is to point out inconsistencies in the literature. Lack of consensus in itself is an important piece of information; it strengthens your argument that further research (your study) is needed.

Summary and Research Gaps

At the end of the literature review, write a brief summary that pulls everything together and highlights the important findings of the literature review. Note any areas where there is little information or conflicting information. In a dissertation, you will then identify the research gaps and make a statement about why it is important to address those gaps. Use a transitional sentence to move into this paragraph, one that clearly connects the "what we know" with the "need to know." For example:

We know this works in that population, but no one has tested it in this population…

We know these things about the topic, but no one has looked at this aspect…

Even though we know that…we haven't examined it in this context…

Despite the evidence of the problems this causes, we've never looked at it from this angle…

Considering the importance of [concept] in other areas, it is time we looked at it in relation to this problem…

SUMMARY EXAMPLE

This literature review provides compelling evidence of the devastating impact of IPV on the lives of the women and the particularly difficult challenges faced by rural women who experience IPV. Women in rural settings must overcome multiple barriers to getting help and leaving an abusive relationship, including isolation, lack of resources, limited access to help, economic constraints, and sociocultural factors (REFERENCES).

Isolation in particular creates multiple hardships for rural women. It limits social support, increases vulnerability, decreases economic opportunities, and makes it difficult to access resources (REFERENCES). In addition, a unique combination of privacy norms and patriarchal attitudes in rural settings can result in a culture of nonintervention (REFERENCES). This is especially concerning because it has been shown that nonintervention norms constrict women's help-seeking behaviors and decreases societal restraints on the violence. Browning (2002) used social disorganization theory to explore the effects of collective efficacy on women's response to IPV. He found that nonintervention norms were associated with higher rates of nonlethal severe IPV, though not intimate-partner homicide, through its effect of lowering collective efficacy and social support in a community. He posited that violent relationships "may remain private (and persist) in part because women perceive their social environment as being unable or unwilling to provide effective social support" (p. 848).

Women's interactions with the healthcare system continue to be problematic. Women report that they will disclose abuse if providers are nonjudgmental, supportive, and knowledgeable (REFERENCES). Yet studies consistently find negative attitudes, discomfort addressing IPV with women, and lack of knowledge among healthcare providers (REFERENCES). Concerns identified by the women in their interactions with the healthcare system, particularly related to safety and confidentiality, take on greater significance in the rural setting where women are isolated, the response of law enforcement may be prolonged, and people are likely to know each other or have relationships in common (REFERENCES) (Roush, 2014).

Note: References in the above excerpt were removed for brevity.

RESEARCH GAPS EXAMPLE

Little recent research looks at the lived experience of IPV in rural women living in the community other than that focused on specific subpopulations or narrow topics. Yet evidence suggests these women face unique and extraordinary challenges associated with IPV. Understanding the lived experience of IPV is crucial in improving outcomes for rural women who experience IPV. Effective programs must be based on the realities of their everyday lives, what resources they believe would be most valuable and how they would use them, and what they see as facilitators and barriers to ending the violence.

WRITING TIP   ORGANIZING YOUR LITERATURE REVIEW

Use sticky notes to help organize sections of your literature review. Each paragraph should have one main idea that can be written in one sentence. Write that main idea for each paragraph in plain language on an individual sticky note and line them up in the order of the paragraphs. Now read through them in order. Does it make sense? Does it flow from one idea to the next? Are there any gaps in the flow of information? Rearrange your sticky notes to optimize the flow, and then move your paragraphs around in the text accordingly.

WRITING TIP   USE MANY SUBHEADINGS

The literature review is likely to be the longest chapter of the dissertation or capstone paper. And you're probably going to cover a lot of different concepts and multiple variables. Subheadings can help you organize the information and can help guide the reader through complex material.

Unfortunately, using lots of headings also makes it hard to keep track of which level of heading you're at, so you can adhere to APA formatting guidelines. For easy reference, write out the heading levels in correct APA formatting (as shown in the following sidebar) in a Word document and print. After you finish the literature review, list all the headings you use in the order you use them in a separate Word document. Then go through and, using your printed list as a guide, assign the appropriate level to each and format it accordingly in the list (capital letters or lowercase, italicized or not, bold or not, ending with a period or not, and so on). Now you can go back to the literature review and make sure that you've got all the headings right.

APA HEADING LEVELS

1	**Centered, Bold, Upper and lowercase**
2	**Flush Left, Bold, Upper and lowercase**
3	**Indented, bold, title case ending with period.**
4	***Indented, bold, italicized, lowercase ending with period.***
5	*Indented, italicized, lowercase ending with a period.*

American Psychological Association (2009). *Publication manual of the American Psychological Association* (6th ed.), p. 62. Washington, D.C: Author.

WRITING TIP   TRANSITIONS

Transitions are particularly important when writing a complex paper that addresses multiple concepts, such as a literature review. Transitions guide the readers through the various ideas and help them understand the connections. Take a few minutes to reread the section on transitions in Chapter 6 for help on creating an organized paper that flows smoothly.

Along with stating what we need to find out or do next, you need to tell us why. Curiosity is not enough; the knowledge/results you are seeking have to serve a purpose. What are the benefits of having this new knowledge? How will this project improve patient outcomes? How will this new understanding help us in providing care? How will it help us improve the healthcare system?

Purpose Statement

This is it. Everything that came before should lead directly to the purpose of your study or project. You've convinced the reader of the importance of your topic. You've summarized what is known and pointed out what is not. Now you tell the reader clearly and concisely what you plan to do next.

Therefore, *I am going to conduct a quality-improvement project to…*

The purpose of this project is to…

Therefore, *I propose a qualitative study to…*

The purpose of this study is to….

If you've done your job well, the reader will be nodding their head in agreement.

Research Questions

Finally, you include your specific research question or questions. This is usually your purpose statement reformulated as a question, but might also include additional questions that drill down into more specifics.

- *What is the lived experience of IPV for women in the context of the rural setting?*

- *What are the IPV-related knowledge, attitudes, beliefs, and behaviors of healthcare providers in the rural setting?*

- *Will biweekly home visits conducted by nurse practitioners for 2 weeks post-hospital discharge reduce readmission rates for heart-failure patients?*

- *Does participation in simulation teamwork exercises improve the perception of teamwork among interprofessional operating room staff?*

If you have specific hypotheses, which is likely if you are doing a quantitative research study, you include those in this section as well.

Now you need to tell readers just how you're going to answer the questions (that is, your methodology), which is the subject of the next chapter.

Chapter Checkup

Did I ...

- ❏ Provide an overview of what is included in the chapter?

- ❏ Establish the scope and severity of the issue?

- ❏ Define all the variables, concepts, and factors?

- ❏ Describe the theoretical model and how it applies to my study?

- ❏ Point out and discuss inconsistencies in the literature?

- ❏ Include a critical appraisal of the research?

- ❏ Include only information directly related to my study or project and clearly show how it's related?

- ❏ Synthesize information rather than list each study separately?

- ❏ Build a strong case for the importance of the topic or issue?

- ❏ Clearly show that my study or project is the logical thing to do?

- ❏ Formulate research questions and hypotheses that are derived from the purpose of the study?

- ❏ Make sure all the citations in the text are in my reference list and vice versa?

Appraisal Tools

Consolidated Criteria for Reporting Qualitative Research (COREQ): COREQ provides a checklist for appraising qualitative research reports.

http://intqhc.oxfordjournals.org/content/19/6/349.long

CONsolidated Standards of Reporting Trials (CONSORT): This group provides a checklist and flow sheet for appraising reports of clinical trials.

http://www.consort-statement.org/consort-2010

Critical Appraisal Skills Programme (CASP): CASP has free tools for appraising different types of research, including systematic reviews and quantitative and qualitative research studies.

http://www.casp-uk.net/#!casp-tools-checklists/c18f8

Preferred Reporting Items for Systematic Reviews and Meta-Analyses (PRISMA): PRISMA provides a checklist and flow sheet for appraising systematic reviews and meta-analyses.

http://www.prisma-statement.org/index.htm

Standards for Quality Improvement Reporting Excellence (SQUIRE): The SQUIRE guidelines provide a checklist for appraising quality improvement projects.

http://squire-statement.org/guidelines

Strengthening the Reporting of Observational Studies in Epidemiology (STROBE): STROBE has free checklists for appraising various types of observational studies.

http://www.strobe-statement.org/index.php?id=available-checklists

References

Roush, K. (2009). Social implications of obstetric fistula: An integrative review. *Journal of Midwifery and Women's Health*, *54*(2), e21–e33. doi: 10.1016/j.jmwh.2008.09.005

Roush, K. (2014). *The experience of intimate partner violence in the context of the rural setting* (Doctoral dissertation, New York University). Available from ProQuest Dissertations and Theses database. (1551746532)

WRITING YOUR METHODOLOGY CHAPTER

ELEMENTS OF YOUR METHODOLOGY CHAPTER

1. Design of the study
2. Setting
3. People involved and resources needed (capstone)
4. Sample, including access and recruitment methods
5. Ethical approvals, including consent
6. How the data will be collected
7. Instruments
8. How data analysis will be conducted
9. How rigor will be ensured
10. Timeline (capstone)
11. Budget (capstone)

This chapter covers how to write up the components of the study's or project's methodology, including the approach, the sample and setting, and procedures of recruitment and data collection. You will also learn what to include regarding instruments and tools used and data management. The chapter ends with a description of how to write up the data analysis.

Chapter Three, the methodology, is where you get down and dirty. It's a detailed account of exactly what you are going to do or, after completing the study or project, what you did. It's actually a pretty straightforward chapter to write because it's very concrete. The key is to be very specific and not miss anything. What you write in your methodology chapter will tell your readers whether your results are valid, reliable, and able to be used with confidence.

Because this is a dissertation or capstone project, you also need to explain why you are doing the study or project this particular way, much more so than if you were writing an article about a study or project. You have to show your professors that you know the rationale behind what you're doing and that each of your choices, from the design to the sampling frame to the statistical method, was a conscious and correct choice.

When you're writing your proposal, everything will be in the future tense. After you finish the study or project and are writing the final paper, you need to return to the methodology chapter and change everything to the past tense.

Explaining the Design of Your Study

The first thing you have to tell the reader is what kind of study or project you are doing and why it is a good fit for your research question. This includes the broader approach of qualitative, quantitative, or mixed methods, and the specific design, such as descriptive, phenomenological, grounded theory, narrative, or ethno-graphic for qualitative studies or experimental, quasi-experimental, or correlational for quantitative research. You can include a little bit of information about how you are going to do it as well.

> *The proposed study will use a descriptive qualitative approach using multiple focus groups of newly licensed RNs working in critical care.*

> *The proposed study will use a quasi-experimental design with electronic surveys administered to participants before and then 6 months following the implementation of the new discharge teaching program.*

You need to provide information about the approach and design that explains why it is the best approach at this time to answer your research question or to address your local problem. You can use expert-authored articles or books on your approach to back up your choices in your methodology chapter.

EXPLANATION OF CHOICE OF APPROACH EXAMPLE

Ethnonursing methodology is very compatible with what this study sought to discover. This method facilitated the discovery and exploration of the meaning of values, beliefs, and health practices of agrarian elders in the rural context from their perspective. The method helped tease out what influence and impact the rural agrarian culture has on the worldview of agrarian elders. In addition, this method helped discover the culture care experiences that have been both helpful and hindering to the well-being of elder agrarians (Witt, 2006)

Some programs might require you to include the theoretical framework or philosophical underpinning in the methodology chapter rather than in the literature review. In that case, it would go here, at the beginning of the chapter.

Establishing Your Study's Setting

Where is your study going to take place? You need to place it within its geographic setting as well as the local (that is, facility or organization) setting if appropriate. Provide enough background information about the setting that the reader understands the context in which the study or problem is taking place. These details might include the population demographics and socioeconomic, environmental, and cultural factors. If the setting is integral to the purpose of the study—for example, a study that looks at a topic specifically related to it happening in a rural area—you will want to include more details.

DESCRIPTION OF SETTING FOR STUDY OF IPV IN A RURAL SETTING

This study was conducted in Warren, Hamilton, and Essex counties in the Adirondack Mountains region of northeastern New York State. All of Hamilton and Essex counties and parts of Warren County meet eligibility requirements for rural health grants according to the Health Resources and Services Administration (HRSA).

Warren County is the southernmost county in the Adirondacks. It covers 867 square miles and has a population of approximately 66,000 people, with one metropolitan area, the city of Glens Falls (U.S. Census Bureau, 2012). The majority of residents are white, 96.8%, with 1% Hispanic, and less than 1% two or more races, African American or American Indian. The median age is 39, and 85% of residents older than 25 have at least a high school diploma, and 23% have at least a bachelor's degree. The median household income from 2006 to 2010 was $51,619, and the average weekly wage was $645, well below the national average of $891 (Bureau of Labor Statistics, 2012; U.S. Census Bureau, 2012). The 2010 estimated number of families living below the poverty level was 1,474 when the householder was female with no husband present compared to 243 when the householder was male with no wife present (U.S. Census Bureau, 2010). (Roush, 2014)

If you are doing a quality-improvement project or a study in a clinical setting, include all the facility or organization information that the reader needs to understand the problem. This includes a description of the organizational culture in addition to information related to administration, management, and nursing leadership structures, financial data, staffing patterns, and patient population. Anything that could influence the implementation or outcomes of your project, for better or worse, should be discussed.

For a capstone project, this is where you are most likely required to describe the people involved in your project. (Again, check your program's specific instructions.) You need to work in partnership with key stakeholders in the organization where the project is taking place:

- Who are these people?

- Who is instrumental in moving implementation of the project forward?

- Who will ensure you have the resources, including staff, that you need to proceed?

- Who will provide access to necessary data (such as admission reports)?

These are just some of the people who might be identified as key stakeholders and onboard from the planning stages.

In addition, for a capstone this is also where you describe what resources are needed to implement the project. This includes human resources, such as increased nursing staff or expert consultants, or material resources, such as access to a simulation lab, computer programs, or patient teaching supplies.

Establishing Your Sample

What population are you drawing your sample from? Who is going to participate in your study or project? How many participants do you need and how are you going to get them? These are the main questions you'll be answering in this section.

Before answering these questions about the sample, you need to first tell us what type of sampling you are going to do, such as convenience, purposive, random, or consecutive. You should also briefly describe the sample design and why you are using that design for your study.

Next you establish your sampling frame, the general population from which you will recruit your participants. So, for the study of IPV in the rural setting, the sampling frame was women living in the Adirondack region of New York State who experienced IPV. For a study of bereaved parents of estranged children, the sampling frame might be parents attending grief support groups in a particular region of the United States.

 When talking about the people who are in a sample for a quantitative study, you usually refer to them as *subjects*. When talking about the people in a qualitative study, you usually refer to them as *participants*.

Then you tell us whom you want to recruit from that population. You need to specify exactly who qualifies to participate. This is done by establishing inclusion and exclusion criteria, similar to what you did to find articles in your literature search for the literature review. If it's not obvious from the study purpose, you also need to explain why you are including or excluding people with those particular traits.

Characteristics that might be part of inclusion and exclusion criteria include the following:

- Demographics (sex, age, educational level, marital status, and so on)
- Presence or absence of an illness or health condition
- Duration of illness or health condition
- Number of years since experiencing phenomenon being studied
- Professional role
- Primary language (English speaking?)
- Literacy
- Previous experience with intervention
- Location

INCLUSION AND EXCLUSION CRITERIA EXAMPLES

The study will include a purposive sample of women in western Uganda who have experienced obstetric fistula. Inclusion criteria are women 18 years of age and older with a vesicovaginal or rectovaginal fistula secondary to prolonged obstructed labor. Exclusion criteria will be women who have had their fistula for longer than 5 years so that the data reflect current sociocultural norms.

The study will use a convenience sample of nurses working on the cardiac care unit. Inclusion criteria are RNs who work full time, have 2 years or more experience on the unit, and provide direct patient care. Exclusion criteria are advanced practice nurses and nurses who are not dedicated staff for the unit (work on other units as well).

COMMON MISTAKE

Exclusion criteria are not the opposite of inclusion criteria. They are applied *after* inclusion criteria. So, if a characteristic is not present in participants that you want to include, you should not list it as part of the exclusion criteria. For example, if one of your inclusion criteria is women between the ages of 18 and 35, do not list women younger than 18 or older than 35 as exclusion criteria because there won't be anyone younger than 18 or older than 35 to exclude.

Noting Sample Size

Now you have to tell your readers how many participants you want to have in your sample. Of course, the answer to this is very different for a quantitative versus a qualitative study.

If you are doing a quantitative study, you not only have to tell us what your sample size will be, but you also have to show how you came up with that number. The reader needs to know that you have enough participants to establish that the study results will have statistical significance. Therefore, you need to tell your readers what formula you used to determine the power of the study and report the *power*, *probability*, and *effect size* calculated and the minimum sample needed to achieve that.

You should also report the expected response rate and provide support, usually based on other studies that used similar sampling frames. And finally, you need to report how much you will increase the final sample size to account for attrition if you are taking into account loss of subjects during the study period. All of these calculations—power, response rate, and attrition—then yield the targeted number of subjects to be recruited.

For a qualitative study, there usually is not a predetermined sample size; you continue to add participants until you get data saturation (that is, you are not finding any new information with further sampling). However, you can give an estimate based on previous studies of the same or similar topic or phenomenon or with similar participants. State why you are not giving an exact number and how you arrived at the estimate. Support this with expert-authored articles or books.

If you're doing focus groups, tell the reader how many groups and how many participants will be in each group. You can give a minimum and maximum rather than an exact number. But remember, nothing in a study is arbitrary, so here also you want to support with evidence, by using expert-authored publications, how you came up with the numbers.

SAMPLE SIZE FOR QUANTITATIVE RESEARCH EXAMPLE

I used G*Power to conduct an a priori power analysis to calculate sample size. For a power of 0.80 with an alpha of 0.05 and a moderate 0.5 effect size, it was determined that a sample of 45 patients was needed. To account for attrition if patients were discharged from the unit during the study period, an additional 15% was added, bringing the total sample needed to 52.

SAMPLE SIZE FOR QUALITATIVE RESEARCH EXAMPLE

Purposive sampling will continue until saturation is reached. Based on a review of the literature of narrative studies in marginalized populations of women (cite studies), the initial estimated sample size is 10 to 15 women. However, due to the uniqueness of individual stories and the emergent process intrinsic to qualitative research, the final sample size cannot be determined until data collection and analysis are underway (cite expert sources).

Describing Recruitment

Finally, you need to describe just how you're going to get the people you need to participate in your study. How are you going to reach people who are eligible to participate? How are you going to ask them to participate? It is very important that you describe your recruitment strategy accurately, because recruitment always involves some ethical issues, particularly around questions of coercion and vulnerability. You must address these directly and clearly in describing your recruitment strategy. For example, in a study involving patients undergoing a limited course of treatment, you might indicate that recruitment was done after treatment was completed so that there was no question of coercion.

> *Waiting until treatment is completed to recruit participants reduces the possibility that patients may feel coerced to participate to receive optimal care.*

In general, you need to address the following when describing recruitment:

- **Delivery of information:** Describe how you will deliver the information about the study to potential participants. You might be using posters, newspaper ads, postal mail, emails, or asking people directly.

- **Where you will recruit:** Describe exactly where the recruitment will take place, including locations where posters or flyers will be placed or handed out and by whom. If you are using mail (postal or electronic), describe how many notices will be sent out and on what schedule.

- **What recruitment methodology used (if any):** If you are following a particular method, such as Dillman's (2007), include that fact with a description of the method and a reference.

DESCRIPTION OF RECRUITMENT STRATEGY EXAMPLE

As suggested by Dillman (2007), there were five contacts with the subjects, including a presurvey email letter sent a week before the email letter with enclosed $5 email gift certificate and a web link to the questionnaire, and three reminder email letters at 2, 4, and 8 weeks from the initial contact with the subjects (Djukic, 2009)

- **Contact information:** Describe how potential participants will get in touch with you.

- **Compensation:** State what compensation participants will receive and why. For example, it might be to cover transportation costs or compensate them for their time or simply as an incentive.

- **Snowballing:** If you plan on using or allowing snowball recruitment, you must include that. This is also called referral sampling; participants refer people they know who meet the criteria into the study.

Sometimes you might face challenges in accessing the population under study. In those cases, you need to describe how you are going to gain access, such as using a facilitator or gatekeeper. If you are conducting a study with a vulnerable population or participation could increase or place participants at risk, describe how you plan to manage that risk during recruitment to protect, to the best of your ability, potential participants.

You need to include a copy of any recruitment materials in the appendix. This includes any email text, letters, posters or flyers, and telephone or in-person scripts.

COMMON MISTAKE

You do not report information on the actual sample (including the final sample size and demographics) that you ended up recruiting in your methodology chapter. Anything you didn't know until after you started conducting the study goes in your results chapter (Chapter Four), not the methodology chapter (Chapter Three).

Ethical Approval and Consent

Now that your readers know who you are recruiting and how, you need to tell them about how you are going to protect your subjects or participants. This information includes review by the appropriate institutional review board or boards and consent of participants or subjects.

If your study includes a vulnerable population, you must include detailed information about how you are going to protect them. The U.S. Department of Health and Human Services, *Part 46, Protection of Human Subjects*, has designated certain populations as particularly vulnerable and requires that you demonstrate that their inclusion in a study is justified and that you have taken additional measures to lower their risk (2014). These populations include the following:

- Children

- Prisoners

- Pregnant women

- Mentally disabled persons

- Economically or educationally disadvantaged persons

In some other situations, participation in a study might place people at increased risk, such as victims of intimate partner violence, so you also need to describe how your procedures are designed to mitigate that risk as much as possible.

> For example, the researcher will place recruitment flyers in area health centers and in public settings such as laundromats, convenience stores, grocery stores, and libraries. As a precaution, the flyer will be titled *Women's Health Study* and will not specify intimate partner violence so that participants will not be put at risk if perpetrators see the flyer. The flyer will include tear-off slips of paper across the bottom of the flyer with the researcher's telephone number. Interested women will be directed to call the researcher at which time the study will be explained in detail.

At the completion of the interview, women will receive information about safety planning based on recommendations of the National Center on Domestic and Sexual Violence. The women will also receive a handout with a list of general women's health resources in the community, such as access to breast and cervical cancer screening services along with the local domestic violence shelter and hotline number. This handout is designed to support women who have told their abusers they are participating in a women's health study while also giving them the hotline number.

Do not wait until you are ready to submit to learn about the institutional review board (IRB) process at your school or organization. Do this *early* in the process. This is particularly important if you are doing anything that involves a vulnerable population, settings outside of the United States, or more than minimal risk to participants. In fact, if that is the case, you should talk directly to someone in IRB about your proposal. You don't want to find out after putting in countless hours and great effort that your study or project is not going to get through IRB or could get stalled in the approval process for an unacceptable amount of time. (It could take many months in complex situations.) If you are doing a study or project in a clinical setting, make sure that you know what the procedures are for both your school and the clinical setting.

Writing a Consent Form

Most institutional review boards have specific language for consent forms. Refer to your school's or organization's IRB website and your program's handbook. In general, it needs to include the following:

- Who is conducting the study, including yourself and your committee members, and their contact information

- Brief introduction of yourself and the study

- Purpose of the study

- What the participant is being asked to do and how long it will take

- A statement that the participant can change her mind, refuse to answer any of the questions, or withdraw from the study at any time

- A statement that her decision to participate or not will not affect treatment where appropriate

- What the risks are to the participant

- What the benefits are to the participant. (Most of the time there are no direct benefits to the participant [incentives or compensation are not benefits], but you can say that it *might* benefit others with similar conditions in the future.)

- Whether their participation in the study will be anonymous or confidential and how that will be accomplished to the best of the researcher's ability

- How long and where information about the study (data) will be kept

- Contact information for the IRB approving the study

You need to include a copy of your consent form in the appendix.

Data Collection

Okay, so now your readers know where you're going to do the study or project, whom you're going to recruit and how, and how you're going to protect those participants. Now it's time to tell your readers how you're going to collect the information you're after: the data. This discussion covers this topic in two separate sections for dissertation research: first for qualitative studies, and then for quantitative studies.

This text then covers what you need to include for a capstone quality-improvement project. This section is where you will tell us exactly what you are going to do and what data you are going to collect to measure the outcomes of your project.

Dissertation Research: Qualitative Data Collection

The two most common methods used to collect data in qualitative studies are interviews and focus groups, and those are what is discussed here.

When describing the data collection, you need to include the following:

- **Interviews:** Who will conduct the interviews and where will they be conducted? If there are interviewers other than the researcher, will they be trained and how? Is there a specific timetable for scheduling interviews? How will the interview proceed? Are the interviews structured or unstructured? If you are doing online interviewing, is it synchronous or asynchronous? How many exchanges will there be with participants, and what is the schedule for them? Will the online interviews take place through a program such as SurveyMonkey or Qualtrics, a video conferencing service such as Skype, or via email exchanges?

- **Focus groups:** Who will conduct the focus groups and where will they be conducted? How many people in each group and how many total groups? Provide an explanation for the size of the groups. Are you going to configure the groups around certain characteristics of the participants? If groups are not homogeneous, explain why, because homogeneous focus groups are considered by many to be optimal.

- **Interview guide or questionnaire:** Describe your interview guide or questionnaire. Are you using a previously tested interview guide or questionnaire? If so, what population and for what purpose was it developed and used? Did you obtain any needed permissions to use it? If you developed the guide or questionnaire yourself, what was it based on (the literature, your theoretical model, a pilot study, etc.)? For unstructured interviews, what is the broad opening question?

- **Pilot interviews:** Are you going to conduct any pilot interviews? What are the specific purposes of the pilot interviews? In the final paper (after conducting the study), you need to include what, if any, changes you made based on the pilot interviews.

- **Audio recording:** Will the interviews or focus groups be recorded? If yes, indicate whether participants will be asked for permission, unless this was a criterion for inclusion. When will the recordings be transcribed (immediately, within a certain time period)? Will you be reviewing all transcriptions or a percentage of the transcriptions for accuracy?

- **Post-interview or post–focus group:** Will there be a debriefing? Will you make notes or do summary sheets after each interview or focus group?

Dissertation Research: Quantitative Data Collection

In quantitative research, data are usually collected and measured using an instrument (or tool), whether it is some type of questionnaire completed by subjects or a tool used by the researcher to gather and organize observed data. You need to describe in detail each instrument you are using in your study and why it is a good measurement tool for your purpose.

You also need to include how the instruments were developed, what studies they have been used in, reliability and validity in prior study populations, and any psychometric testing that was done specifically for your study and the results. If you are adapting an instrument for use in your study, you need to describe exactly what was changed and why. State whether permission to use a preexisting instrument was required and, if so, that you received it and from whom.

COMMON MISTAKE

Make sure to report reliability and validity in *your* study population. If the instrument has not been used in similar populations in prior studies, you need to conduct tests to establish reliability and validity with your population.

- **Questionnaires/Surveys:** You need to describe questionnaires in detail. What are the questions trying to get at? What type of questions (Likert-type, multiple-choice, dichotomous, forced-choice, and so on) are there and how many? How is the questionnaire structured and formatted?

  How will the questionnaire or survey be distributed? Will you be using an electronic survey program like SurveyMonkey or Qualtrics? If yes, you need to describe how subjects will move through the instrument, including how many screens and whether subjects will be able to skip screens or move backward and forward. How will you ensure that each person completes the instrument only one time?

- **Observations:** Describe the instrument you are using to record your observations and the protocols for data collection. If more than one person is doing the observations, how are you going to address inter-rater reliability? Are observations being recorded, via either audio or video?

- **Biophysiologic:** You need to report what tests are being done and by whom. Be precise in describing protocols. What equipment will be used to collect the data, and how will accuracy and precision be ensured? If a laboratory is being used to analyze urine or blood samples, you need to establish the normal values for that laboratory.

- **Pilot testing:** Are you going to conduct any pilot testing of the instruments? If yes, who will participate in the pilot testing? What in particular are you looking to learn from the pilot testing? In the final paper, after the study is completed, you will have to describe the results of the pilot testing and any changes that were made based on those results.

General Elements Needed for Qualitative and Quantitative Data Collection

In addition to the elements previously discussed in this chapter, you need to address the following regardless of the type of study or project you are doing:

- **Demographic data:** What demographic data will be collected and at what point in the study? Will it be done before or after the interview or questionnaire or survey is completed?

- **Privacy:** How will the participant's privacy be protected? How will anonymity be achieved? For example, names and any other identifying information will be redacted from recordings or transcripts.

- **Storage:** Where will the data, both audio recordings and transcripts, be kept? How will it be secured for privacy's sake? How long will it be kept before being destroyed?

Capstone Project

In the methodology chapter (or section) of a capstone project, you need to take the reader through the planning of the project, describe in detail the implementation procedures, and provide a timeline and budget:

- **Planning:** Who was involved in the planning and what were their roles? Was a committee formed? Who were the members and what were their responsibilities? Was any kind of a needs assessment done? What resources are needed, and how are you going to get them? Did you create a marketing strategy or develop a business plan? Tell us about any challenges that you expect to encounter and how you plan to address them.

CHALLENGES AND PLAN TO ADDRESS EXAMPLE

Other barriers included existing time pressures and scheduling demands for primary care providers. Given the number of patients scheduled on a daily basis, practice managers expressed a need to keep the program limited to no greater than 90 minutes, and each required sufficient advance notice to schedule a date and time that would allow for all practice providers and staff to attend during office hours. This would limit financial implications such as avoiding paying overtime for hours outside of regular working hours. With this in mind, scheduling was adjusted for each practice setting to allow for the program to be delivered during office hours (Surreira, 2014).

   If there are written agreements with the organization or stakeholders, include a copy in the appendix.

- **Implementation:** This is the nitty-gritty of the project. You need to give your readers a detailed step-by-step account of what you are going to do. You should include all the information needed to replicate your project in another facility or organization. If an educational program is part of the project, include detailed information about the content and delivery method.

You also need to tell us how you are going to know whether your project was successful:

- What outcomes will be measured and how?

- What data are you collecting prior to initiation of the project?

- Are data coming from a public performance reporting survey, such as the Hospital Consumer Assessment of Healthcare Providers and Systems (HCAHPS)?

- When there are training or educational initiatives, will participants complete a pretest and post-test?

- Are you doing a chart review and, if so, how many charts and over what period of time?

REMEMBER

Details! You have all the little ins and outs in your head, and it's easy to skip over what seems inconsequential to you. Read your methodology chapter (section) for gaps and fill them in. Try to anticipate questions. Better yet, have nurses working elsewhere read your methodology and tell you what's missing for them to be able to implement the project at their facility.

Timeline and Budget

You need to include a timeline of the project, beginning with the planning stages and going through evaluation of outcomes. You usually do this in a table format, though you can also use a flow chart or list. Here is a sample timeline.

Completion Date	Planning	Pre-Implementation	Implementation	Evaluation
10/1/2014	Meet with key stakeholders individually to obtain their support			
10/7/2014	First planning meeting			
10/14/2014	Meet with Ed. Dept. to develop educational sessions			
10/15/2014		Begin tracking of CAUTIs on unit		
10/25/2014		Submit IRB application		
10/21/2015	Meet with IT Dept. re: adding CAUTI Alert screen			
10/31/2014		Pilot test CAUTI Alert Screen (not activated)		
4/15/2015		End tracking of CAUTIs on unit		
4/15/2015 to 4/30/2015			Conduct educational sessions on unit	Pretest and post-test of educational sessions
4/15/2015			Place posters on units	

Completion Date	Planning	Pre-Implementation	Implementation	Evaluation
4/15/2015			Activate CAUTI Alert screen on computer	
4/30/2015				Begin tracking use of CAUTI Alert screen
4/30/2015				Begin tracking CAUTIs on unit
10/30/2015				End tracking of CAUTIs on unit
10/30/2015				Survey nurses on perception of CAUTI Alert screen

You also need to provide a budget. Include estimated costs in the proposal and final costs after completing the project, with an explanation of any major discrepancies between the two. Costs might include labor costs to pay nurses for time spent in educational meetings or extra staffing to cover the nurses while they are off the floor for the meetings, educational materials for staff or patients, computer software programs, lab tests, and equipment.

BUDGET EXAMPLE

The budget for the implementation in this QI project has few expenses. The main anticipated expense for hospital resources was the time for the staff deployed to assist the Doctor of Nursing Practice (DNP) candidate extract and process the relevant patient information from the electronic medical records. A clinical informatics consultant already employed by the hospital was consulted as needed on a no-cost basis; however, the cost to the hospital of this service was approximated at $1,360. The DNP candidate volunteered to work full time (40 h per week) to implement the project, but did not expect to receive any pro rata payment for his services.

The only direct incurred cost to the hospital ($450) was for the DNP candidate to organize and conduct seminars to train physicians and other staff and to purchase miscellaneous materials (see Appendix D) (Blake, 2014).

Data Analysis

In the previous sections, you told your readers what data you planned to collect and how and by whom. Now you need to tell your readers how you are going to analyze those data.

There are a number of approaches to be taken in qualitative data analysis and different types of statistics that can be run on quantitative data. Of course, you've already determined which approach you're going to use based on your research question and theoretical framework or philosophical underpinning. Here you're going to explain the mechanics.

 When you are writing your proposal, this section will be in the future tense. After you complete data collection, you will need to go back and change it to the past tense.

Qualitative Data Analysis

Begin with a general statement about the approach you are taking, and describe briefly how data analysis is done when using that approach. Talk about the ongoing iterative process; that analysis begins in the field and will inform data collection as it proceeds, including refining questionnaires or interview guides for subsequent interviews. Provide expert-authored resources to support your choices and the process.

There are a number of different approaches to analysis of qualitative data depending on the type of study and method. If you are following a recognized researcher's method, such as Creswell, describe the step-by-step process for analysis. This often will include some or all of the following in a similar order:

- Immersion in the data
- Reading the text of the interviews or focus groups through the lens of the research question or theoretical framework
- Constant comparison
- Coding
- Alternating between parts and the whole
- Repeating the process
- Identification of themes and patterns

It might help to give an example of coding.

Tell us how you will know when coding is completed. Will there be additional coders? Where in the process will they be involved, and what percentage of the data will they analyze?

Will you do a member check? How will that be done, and how many of the participants will be asked? If there is a member check, you need to make a statement about the feedback in your final paper.

State whether you are using a software program, such as ATLAS.ti or NVivo, to analyze the data or whether you will doing it manually.

DESCRIPTION OF DATA ANALYSIS EXAMPLE

Data analysis followed processes outlined by Creswell (2007). I began with immersion in the data, reading and rereading the entire text of interviews and field notes several times and making notes. Constant comparison was then done to code data, comparing all the pieces of data against each other and against the text in its entirety. For example, if women stated that there were no nearby neighbors, that the closest town was out of reach, or that they did not have transportation to go visit family, it would be coded as isolation. Or if women stated that their family tells them to accept the violence to stay in the relationship or their neighbors refuse to help, it would be coded as lack of support. After I did initial coding, a second coder read and assigned initial codes to 20% of the data, and then she and I sat together and went through the interviews to challenge the coding (Roush, 2014).

Quantitative Data Analysis

It's hard to imagine nowadays how researchers managed quantitative data analysis without the statistical software programs that are available to us. Now all we have to do is plug in our data and click on the appropriate tabs and *voilà*! In a matter of seconds, we are presented with the results we need.

Of course, it's not quite that simple. The programs can't tell us what tests to run in the first place or why. That's where your critical thinking and research knowledge come in. And that's what you are going to explain in detail here.

- **Type of statistical analysis:** Begin by stating the type of statistical analysis you will be performing and what you have set for your alpha value. State whether you are using a statistical software program such as Statistical Package for the Social Sciences (SPSS) or the Statistical Analysis System (SAS).

> Path analysis was used to construct a model identifying significant predictors of the major dependent variable (QOL). Bivariate correlation measures were performed to determine what relationships, if any, exist between the independent variables. An alpha of 0.05 was used for all statistical tests in this study (Hay, 2005).
>
> I will perform descriptive analysis of the data, including frequency distribution, dispersion, and measures of central tendency.
>
> Bivariate inferential statistical analysis will include independent t-tests and multiple linear regression.

- **Coding:** Describe the coding scheme that you used and who did the coding. If more than one person coded, did you assess intercoder reliability and how? Include the coding instructions and codebook in the appendices. Was any recoding of data done? If you used a Likert scale, will you do reverse coding for negatively worded items?

  If you are using a Likert-type scale, you also need to describe the scale, including whether there is a neutral response (if not, you should explain why, because it is generally considered best to include one) and the strength and direction of the choices. What is the range of possible scores for the complete scale?

- **Preliminary analysis:** Describe any preliminary analyses that will be done. This includes data cleaning for code errors, missing values, and outliers. In the final paper, tell your readers what values were missing, any patterns or rationale for them, and what strategy you used to deal with them.

How will you determine whether there is normal distribution of the variables, in addition to other assumptions, for inferential tests? Describe what possible biases (nonresponse bias, for instance) you looked for in the data and how that was done. If there is a question of bias, how did you address it?

If you do find evidence of biases, you do not discuss them in the methodology chapter (Chapter Three). Instead, you do so in the discussion chapter (Chapter Five) when you talk about study limitations.

- **Analysis:** Finally, describe in detail each type of analysis that was done in the order that it was done for each of the variables or for each hypothesis. If you are doing any multiple regression analysis, state in what order the variables were entered into the equation.

Rigor

By now, your readers have a good idea of how rigorous your study is based on everything you've told them about your methodology. However, there are measures that are taken, whether for qualitative or quantitative research, that are specifically meant to enhance the rigor of the study. This last part of your methodology chapter will describe these for the reader.

Qualitative

There continues to be debate about how to assess rigor, or even if you can, in qualitative research, so it's important to acknowledge and briefly discuss this in the beginning of this section. You should cite expert-authored texts for this discussion. If you are following a particular expert's framework, such as Lincoln and Guba (1985), state that and structure your discussion by the relevant criteria.

At the minimum, tell your readers how you will establish trustworthiness and credibility. Possible measures that should be described include the following:

- Triangulation
- Engaging in reflexivity
- Prolonged engagement
- Looking for disconfirming evidence or negative cases
- Keeping an audit trail
- Using thick description and verbatim quotes
- Doing a member check
- Using an independent coder
- Getting peer review

Quantitative

In quantitative research, you need to convince the reader of the reliability, validity, and generalizability of your study. Much of this is related to how you sample and the instruments you use. Using instruments that have been shown to be valid and reliable in your population, whether in previous studies or through pyschometric testing you perform, is critical, and you should talk about that here, even though you included information on it earlier. You should also describe how your sampling and recruitment techniques will help avoid potential bias and increase generalizability.

Congratulations! You've reached an important milestone: The proposal for your dissertation or capstone project is done! You are now ready to defend it. After that, you'll get IRB approval, and then on to the fun stuff: data collection.

Then, after you've collected all your data, onward to the next chapter/section, results.

Chapter Checkup

❑ Did I clearly explain why I chose the study design?

❑ Is the intervention described in enough detail for others to replicate it?

❑ Is the sampling method described?

❑ Are the sample exclusion and inclusion criteria clear?

❑ Did I report validity and reliability of the instruments being used?

❑ Have I described the resources needed for a quality-improvement project?

❑ Did I describe ethical considerations and IRB approval?

❑ Have I provided enough information about the coding scheme?

❑ Have I described preliminary analyses, including tests of assumption for inferential statistics?

❑ Have I described in detail each statistical test being done?

❑ Have I included copies of the following in the appendix: consent forms, recruitment materials, interview guides, surveys, and instruments/tools?

References

Blake, J. (2014). *Improving the transition of care from the hospital to primary care providers for patients with heart failure* (Doctor of nursing practice [DNP] capstone project, University of Massachusetts Amherst). Retrieved from http://scholarworks.umass.edu/nursing_dnp_capstone/38/

Dillman, D. A. (2007). *Mail and internet surveys: The tailored design method.* New York, NY: Wiley

Djukic, M. (2009). *Physical work environment: Testing an expanded job satisfaction model in a sample of hospital staff registered nurses* (Doctoral dissertation, New York University). Available from ProQuest Dissertations and Theses database. (3382425)

Hay, C. G. (2005). *Predictors of quality of life of elderly end-stage renal disease patients: An application of Roy's model* (Georgia State University). Retrieved from ProQuest Dissertations and Theses, http://search.proquest.com/docview/304999693?accountid=27880. (304999693)

Lincoln, Y. S., & Guba, E. G. (1985). *Naturalistic inquiry.* Beverly Hills, CA: Sage.

Roush, K. (2014). *The experience of intimate partner violence in the context of the rural setting* (Doctoral dissertation, New York University). Available from ProQuest Dissertations and Theses database. (1551746532)

Surreira, C. (2014). *Culturally competent LGBT care* (Doctor of nursing practice [DNP] capstone project, University of Massachusetts Amherst). Retrieved from http://scholarworks.umass.edu/nursing_dnp_capstone/34

U.S. Department of Health and Human Services. (2014). *Code of Federal Regulations, Part 46, Protection of human subjects.* Retrieved from http://www.hhs.gov/ohrp/humansubjects/guidance/45cfr46.html

Witt, D. E. (2006). *Growing old on the farm: An ethnonursing examination of aging and health within the agrarian rural subculture* (Doctoral dissertation, Duquesne University). Available from ProQuest Dissertations and Theses database.

Resources

Creswell, J. W. (2007). *Qualitative inquiry and research design: Choosing among five traditions.* Thousand Oaks, CA: Sage Publications.

Creswell, J. W., & Miller, D. L. (2000). Determining validity in qualitative inquiry. *Theory into Practice, 39*(3), 124–130.

Mays, N., & Pope, C. (1995). Qualitative research: Observational methods in health care settings. *British Medical Journal, 311*(6998), 182–184.

Miles, M. B., & Huberman, A. (1994). *Qualitative data analysis: An expanded sourcebook.* Thousand Oaks, CA: Sage.

Polit, D. F., & Beck, C. T. (2012). *Nursing research: Principles and methods* (9th ed.). Philadelphia, PA: Lippincott, Williams, & Wilkins.

Polkinghorne, D. E. (2007). Validity issues in narrative research. *Qualitative Inquiry, 13*(4), 471–486.

Pope, C., Ziebland, S., & Mays, N. (2000). Analyzing qualitative data. *British Medical Journal, 320*(7227), 114–116.

Sandelowski, M. (1995). Sample size in qualitative research. *Research in Nursing & Health, 18*(2), 179–183.

Vanden Bosch, M. (2011). *Comparative analysis of the demographic, clinical, and social-cognitive factors associated with physical activity among middle-aged women with and without diabetes* (Doctoral dissertation, Michigan State University). Available from ProQuest Dissertations and Theses database. (916256697)

WRITING YOUR
RESULTS CHAPTER

ELEMENTS OF YOUR RESULTS
CHAPTER

1. Response rate

2. Final sample size

3. Demographics with descriptive statistics

4. Results of preliminary statistical tests that
    were performed

5. Results of all final statistical analyses that
    were done

6. Outcomes of project evaluation in a
    capstone project

This chapter covers how to write up your results. The chapter covers writing up quantitative and qualitative results and the evaluation of a capstone project.

Congratulations! You've finished collecting your data and analyzing it or have fully implemented your quality-improvement (QI) project. Now you have to tell your readers what you found or how successful the project was. If you did a quantitative study, this is usually fairly straightforward and standardized. It can get a little more complicated for QI projects when you have results across multiple phases to report on. And it can get even more complicated in qualitative research, when you can have hundreds of pages of interview data to sift through to decide what to include in your results section/chapter.

First you want to go back and change all the wording on data analysis to past tense. It's no longer something you're going to do; it's something you did (feels good, right?).

The most important thing to keep in mind as you write up your results is that you are *only reporting the results* in this chapter. You *are not interpreting or discussing them.* That comes in the Discussion chapter.

Begin as usual with a short paragraph describing what you are going to cover in this chapter.

EXAMPLE OF INTRODUCTION TO RESULTS CHAPTER

This chapter presents the results of the data analysis, including the quantitative survey results and answers to the open-ended qualitative questions. Demographics are described and key findings highlighted.

Results

In reporting your results, follow your process of analysis and build a case as you answer each research question or address each aim or hypothesis of your study. You are logically leading the reader to the conclusions that you will present in the discussion chapter.

You should provide the dates of data collection. What dates were the survey open? Over what period of time did interviews take place? What were the date parameters for chart reviews? For a QI project, give dates for both data collection before implementation, dates of implementation, and dates for data collection after implementation.

The following subsections outline a way to organize the findings under subheads commonly needed in reporting results. Remember, though, to always check your specific program's guidelines.

Preliminary Analyses

Report the results of any preliminary analyses you completed and actions taken as a result (change in statistical test performed, items deleted or added, changes made to instruments, variables excluded from analysis). Provide details on missing values and how you dealt with them. When using multiple instruments, you could report the psychometric results for all of them in a paragraph upfront or report on each when you present the results of the analysis that was done using that instrument.

Describe the results of the tests you ran to check that assumptions were met for each of the statistical tests you used. You can do this in the text by simply stating which tests of assumptions were met and which were not. You could also include histograms or probability plots in your paper that support your statements. Provide a reference for cutoff values. For example, if you considered a skew ratio greater than 2 as the cutoff for normal distribution, provide the rationale and cite an expert-authored source to support it. If assumptions were not met, you need to give more details, including how you addressed it.

In a qualitative study, you need to report the results of any pilot tests you did on your interview guide or questionnaire, along with any changes that were made based on the pilot tests. Also, because of the iterative nature of qualitative research, where data analysis begins with data collection and can create the need for method-ological changes along the way, you must report on any adjustments you made to the method from how it was originally described in your proposal and what triggered those adjustments.

EXAMPLE OF REPORT OF CHANGES DUE TO PILOT TESTING

I began with a scripted introduction of the study followed by general questions about IPV in the local community. In initial interviews, the interviewer then asked structured questions to elicit an exploration of the participant's experiences.

Two pilot interviews were conducted to get a better estimate of how long the interviews would take and to see whether there were any unforeseen difficulties with any of the questions. Based on these interviews, I changed the interview approach to more of a narrative format. The interviewer asked participants to tell their story and asked for clarification or more details. When participants finished telling their story, I returned to the interview guide to ensure that all questions had been addressed. The interviews were transcribed, and I reviewed all transcriptions, checking accuracy against the recording (Roush, 2014).

Response Rate

You should state what the response rate was in sample recruitment and how it was calculated. How many of the surveys returned were incomplete? Did nonresponders differ at all from responders? Did anyone leave a focus group or decline to continue after starting an interview? Were any adjustments made in recruitment based on early response rates?

Sample Size and Demographics

State your final sample size and the numbers in any subgroups. If participants were recruited from different types of settings that could have a meaningful effect on results (an acute-care hospital and a long-term care facility, for example), tell your readers how many were from each setting. You may report the final sample size and response rate together if there were no special considerations, such as a disproportionate response rate from a particular subgroup. Describe in the text any demographics that are relevant to the meaning of the study, and include a table with descriptive statistics of all the sample demographics.

EXAMPLE OF REPORT OF RESPONSE RATE, SAMPLE SIZE, AND DEMOGRAPHICS

A total of 108 advanced practice nurses (APNs) responded to the survey for a response rate of 52%. Ten of the surveys were not completed, and these were removed from analysis, leaving a final sample size of 98 APNs. Adult nurse practitioners represent the highest proportion of respondents (58%), followed by gerontological nurse practitioners (32%). Most were female (88%) and white (89%), and between 30 and 59 years of age. Sample demographics are in Table 1. Among the 94 APNs who responded to the question on practice setting, physician-owned private practice and long-term care facilities (LTCF) were the most represented clinical practice areas (n=44 and n=27, respectively).

Report aggregate demographics for each characteristic; do not list demographic information for each participant. You don't want to compromise confidentiality by unintentionally providing identifying information.

COMMON MISTAKE

Be consistent in reporting. For example, if you report standard deviation from the mean for one set of descriptive data, you need to report it for all. Use the same number of decimal places for all numbers (usually two).

Findings

Provide a general statement of the results for each hypothesis or statistical test that was done and specific details that you think should be highlighted. You can point out items in a Likert scale that had the highest and lowest scores, the factors with the highest or lowest frequency, what significant correlations were found and their intensity (weak, moderate, strong), and important negative findings. Include the tests of statistical significance that were used and the values (alpha, chi square, or confidence interval) in parentheses after each result. All the detailed results should then be in tables.

When reporting results, make sure that the reader has the information to know what they mean. For example, in a Likert scale, you must indicate what the values for each item represent.

EXAMPLE OF DESCRIPTION OF LIKERT SCALE

Attitudes and beliefs were measured with 5-point Likert scale questions with a range from 1 = strongly disagree to 5 = strongly agree, including a middle neutral option. Mean scores above the midpoint of 2.5 reflect more favorable or objective attitudes or beliefs, whereas those below 2.5 indicate less-favorable or less-objective attitudes or beliefs (Roush, 2014).

Don't Just Throw a Lot of Data at Us!

Make sure that each result being reported is logical and meaningful to your study. This is where critical thinking and discrimination come into play. Just because SPSS or SAS spits out a table doesn't mean it necessarily belongs in your paper. When you did the analysis, for example, you might have found results that were not related to your research question or hypotheses. They should not be included in your results. (They might be something to consider for another study.) However, you do want to include relevant negative findings. After all, knowing what doesn't work can be as important as knowing what does.

This is true for qualitative results, as well, and perhaps even more so. Your data will include a tremendous number of quotations. You want to pull out and include those that *best* represent the results, not just give readers an endless litany of quotations. For more on this, see the section on qualitative results later in this chapter.

You could also include a diagram of your theoretical framework from earlier in the paper and insert key findings in the appropriate areas (see Figure 4.1). This will not work with all theoretical frameworks, but when it does, it can be a nice way of illustrating the operational application of the framework as you carried out the study.

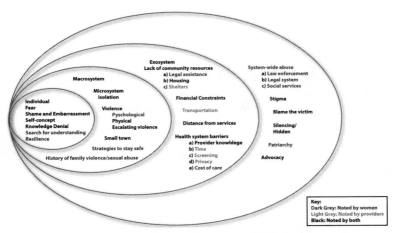

Figure 4.1   Theoretical model illustration with findings inserted

Tables and Figures

Tables list and tabulate results, and figures provide a visual representation of data. Figures are great for illustrating *trends or patterns*. For example, if you want to show the changing rate of CAUTIs on your unit over the duration of your quality-improvement project, a graph will do that much better than a list of numbers in a table (see Figure 4.2). If you just want to show the difference between the rate at the beginning and the rate after implementation, a table is the better choice (see Table 4.1).

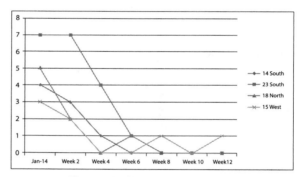

Figure 4.2   Number of new CAUTIs

Table 4.1   Number of New CAUTIs

Unit	January 2014	April 2014
14 South	4	0
23 South	7	0
18 North	5	0
15 West	3	1

In a quantitative study, you will likely have numerous tables in the results chapter/section. You will include the major findings and any other findings you think should be highlighted in the text, but you'll present many of the results of the statistical tests in table form. One way to determine what belongs in the text is whether you plan to talk about it in the discussion chapter; if so, you should report it in the text, not just in a table. You will usually embed tables in the text close to where you refer to them. As always, though, check the requirements of your program; some might want all the tables placed in an appendix (although you will still refer to the table by number in the text and refer reader to the appendix).

 Pie graphs are rarely a good choice for representing statistical results. They are just not precise enough. Avoid them.

You can combine factors or characteristics in a table when there are relatively few in each group and when such a combination of factors will not affect reader understanding or the meaning of results. For example, if you are reporting on comorbidities in patients with heart failure and a large proportion of patients have lung disease, diabetes, anemia, and renal insufficiency, and just a few have one of a dozen other conditions, you would list lung disease, diabetes, anemia, and renal insufficiency in their own rows or columns, and then collapse the others into an Other row or column. There is no hard and fast number for when you would collapse a category; it depends on the overall sample size and the average size of the groups. If there are 10 or 20 in a group, you might want to collapse those with less than 5, but if there are hundreds of participants in each group, you might combine groups that have only 10 or 20.

Be sure to highlight statistically significant findings for the reader. You do this by placing an asterisk (*) next to significant p values in the body of the table and a key at the bottom. One asterisk is used for *p = 0.05, and two asterisks are used for **p = 0.01.

Do not just automatically transpose the output from SPSS or SAS as your tables. Some will work fine as is, but you should also create your own tables from the results or revise where needed to present the results in a way that best addresses your research questions and enhances your readers' understanding.

Refer to the appropriate formatting guide (most likely APA) for how to construct tables. General rules include the following:

- Each table must be able to stand alone. That means that you must spell out acronyms and explain symbols even if they've already been used in the text or another table.

- Be consistent in style across tables.

- Use a legend or key to explain symbols or abbreviations.

Qualitative Results

Writing up qualitative results is challenging. You might have hundreds of pages of data from interviews even after you complete coding. The specific mechanics of how you write up your qualitative results will depend first on the type of qualitative research you did and second on the analysis method you are following. However, some guidelines cut across all the approaches. For the most part, you will be telling a story, and the data you collected and the quotations and observations are the building blocks of that story; they shape and support it.

You can organize your paper by the themes you identified. Start with a general statement about the findings and list the themes and sub-themes that you identified in your analysis. Then using a sub-head for each theme, provide detailed findings for each with the supporting data (such as quotes and observations).

EXAMPLE OF ARRANGING FINDINGS BY THEMES

The participants all described a complex web of intersecting factors at all levels of the ecological model; from internal struggles with self-identity at the individual level and abuses of power and control in relationships at the microsystem level as well as at the macrosystem and exosystem levels. They all also described efforts to prevail over the abuse they suffered and multiple barriers they encountered in trying to create a life separate from the abuser. The result is a picture of isolated lives circumscribed by violence and efforts to stay safe while at the same time engaged in a dynamic search for understanding and eventually a better life.

Six major themes were identified:

1. *Living with violence,* which describes the participants' relationship with the abuser and the day-to-day experience of abuse and includes sub-themes of history of childhood abuse, taken by surprise, physical abuse, psychological abuse, substance abuse, and impact of physical violence

2. *Protect self,* which describes the participants' efforts to decrease the abuse and stay safe

3. *Isolation,* which describes the isolating factors associated with the abuse and includes sub-themes of social isolation, small town, and stigma

4. *Search for understanding,* which describes the participants' efforts to understand their situation

5. *System level abuse,* which describes the role of community and societal factors, and includes sub-themes blame the victim, law enforcement, and legal system

6. *Creating a new life,* which describes the participants' efforts to escape the abuse and create a better life for themselves and, where applicable, their children and includes sub-themes of on-again, off-again; finally "done"—leaving for good; finding support; making it on their own; the abuse still just continues—staying safe; and "I'll be alright. It'll just take time"—resilience and recovery.

Following is a detailed description of each of the themes and sub-themes with supporting data.

(Roush, 2014)

How many quotations should you include in your paper? The answer: There is no set number. You need to include enough quotations—and the right quotations—to support your results in a way that causes readers to trust those results. This is called *thick description*, and it is one of the ways you show the rigor of your study and convince the reader that your results are reliable. One or two quotations do not establish a theme. However, you do not want to list every quotation that resulted in a theme or a pattern being established. Choose the quotations that most powerfully demonstrate the theme or pattern being presented. Some quotations can be interwoven into the text, and others can be separated from the body of the text.

EXAMPLE OF PRESENTATION OF QUOTATIONS

Respondents had mixed views about the overall attitude of the community, with some statements reflecting the view of one respondent who wrote, "The community does not condone abuse," and others expressing opinions more in line with the respondent who wrote that it "is generally accepted by the community."

> *I feel they have mixed views; some people aware of a problem will try to help when they can, and others will look the other way.*

> *I think the prevailing views are it's unfortunate and there is help in the community if someone can help you reach out* (Roush, 2014).

Be precise when writing the quotations from participants. Do not embellish or amplify. When face-to-face interviews were conducted, note interviewee nonverbal expressions of emotions that the reader needs to be aware of to have a full and accurate understanding of what is being conveyed by the participant. This might include facial expressions, such as smiles or grimaces; laughter or crying; and physical actions such as clenching their fists, hiding their face, and shaking or nodding their head.

You can remove words that are extraneous if doing so doesn't change the meaning, and you can add words for context or understanding, again so long as it doesn't change the meaning. However, you have to indicate that you have done so by using an ellipsis (…) where you have removed words and brackets ([ ]) around words you've added.

It also helps to provide context for some of the quotations by adding information about the participant or the situation. This can add depth to the report of the findings. Be careful, though, that you are not compromising confidentiality by adding identifying information or too many details about a participant's situation. You might need to give a general rather than specific age and redact dates or places in the description or in the quote itself.

EXAMPLE OF ADDING CONTEXT TO QUOTATIONS

One of the participants, a woman in her early 20s who had left her husband 6 months prior to the focus group, talked about an earlier attempt she made to leave her marriage.

> *I left him in [year] for 8 or 9 months and got an apartment out by [town] with just the baby and me, but he would come over, then call three, four, five times a day begging us to come back. So I went back to him. Cause I was trying to work and take care of the baby and all. And then being harassed on top of everything. It was easier to go back than to deal with it.*

Avoid the use of adjectives. Let the power of the participants' words convey emotion and intensity. And remember, you are presenting *data,* so you don't want to unduly influence the reader's response to it by telling them how to think or feel about it.

Remember, the quotations are the *data*. They are not the results. The results, depending on the type of qualitative study you're doing, are the synthesis, themes, patterns, or theories that come from analyzing the quotations. When writing, you state the results and then add the quotations—the data—that support the results.

Finally, *give yourself plenty of time*. Writing up qualitative results is time-consuming if you are going to do it well. You will need to go back and revise, again and again, adding in quotations, taking others out, and moving things around, to arrive at the composition that best tells the story of your results. Get feedback from your committee or other qualitative researchers as you work.

Capstone Project Evaluation and Outcomes

The evaluation of a capstone is a detailed report of how the implementation process proceeded, step by step, as well as the outcomes. What happened after you started the intervention? Describe the facilitators and barriers you encountered and what adjustments you made as a result. What about unintended consequences?

Describe incremental outcomes that were measured and what, if any, actions were taken as a result. Use a graph to show changes over time and note on the graph when particular actions were taken (see Figure 4.3). Use tables to present results of quantitative measurements that were done (see Table 4.2).

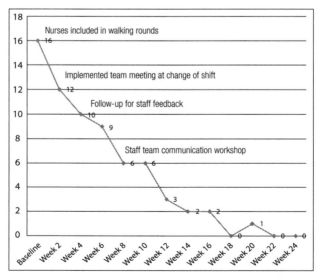

Figure 4.3   Number of Shift Hand-off Problems.

Table 4.2 Types of Hand-off Problems

	Base-line	Weeks post-implementation											
		2	4	6	8	10	12	14	16	18	20	22	24
Admission or discharge delays	2	3	2	4	3	3	2	1	1	0	0	0	0
Medications not given	2	2	1	0	0	0	0	0	0	0	0	0	0
Medical orders not received	1	0	0	1	0	0	0	0	0	0	0	0	0
Care not documented	1	2	1	1	0	0	0	1	0	0	0	0	0
Family member communication missed	3	2	1	2	1	2	1	0	1	0	1	0	0
Change in patient status not updated	2	1	2	0	1	0	0	0	0	0	0	0	0
Concerns not communicated	3	1	2	1	1	1	0	0	0	0	0	0	0
Missed Care	2	1	1	0	0	0	0	0	0	0	0	0	0
Total	16	12	10	9	6	6	3	2	2	0	1	0	0

If you find it difficult to organize all the moving parts of your project evaluation, think about the write-up in a Plan-Do-Study-Act (PDSA) framework. You might have used this framework for your project to begin with, so reporting the Do-Study-Act of each phase is straightforward. Even if you didn't follow this framework, though, you can use it as a writing tool to help you organize all the pieces of information of the project in a clear, easy-to-follow structure and ensure that you're covering everything you need to cover. The pre-implementation data and activities are the (Plan) aspect of this framework. You then report on the initial implementation (Do) and the early evaluation (Study), including any data you had collected at that point and outcomes such as responses from staff or patients, challenges you encounter, and unforeseen complications. Tell your readers about adjustments you made in response to those outcomes (Act). Repeat this sequence as often as needed to describe all the activities and interim evaluations of the project period.

Ensure that the final outcomes pertain directly to the problem statement and the purpose of the project as you stated it in your introduction chapter (Chapter One). And go back through your goals and aims and make sure that you've addressed each of them in the evaluation as well.

Okay, now that you've finished telling your readers what your study found or what happened with your project, you now need to tell them what it all means.

Chapter Checkup

❏ Are findings clearly and logically organized?

❏ Are graphics (tables, figures, graphs) used appropriately?

❏ Are readers able to understand tables and graphs without having to refer back to the text?

❏ Did I describe the final sample and any sub-groups?

❏ Did I provide a summary of the demographics?

❏ Did I present the findings without interpretation or comments on their implications?

❏ Did I include all relevant results and only relevant results?

❏ Was I consistent in how I reported statistical results?

❏ Did I protect the confidentiality of participants in writing up interview results?

❏ Did I address each of the research questions or hypotheses?

❏ Are the outcomes of my project directly related to the problem statement?

❏ Did I address all the goals and objectives of the project?

References

Roush, K. (2014). *The experience of intimate partner violence in the context of the rural setting* (Doctoral dissertation., New York University). Available from ProQuest Dissertations and Theses database. (1551746532)

Resources

Creswell, J. W. (2007). *Qualitative inquiry and research design: Choosing among five traditions.* Thousand Oaks, CA: Sage Publications.

Institute for Healthcare Improvement. (2011). *How to improve.* Retrieved from http://www.ihi.org/resources/Pages/HowtoImprove/default.aspx

Lincoln, Y. S., & Guba, E. G. (1985). *Naturalistic inquiry.* Newbury Park, CA: Sage Publications.

Miles, M. B., & Huberman, A. (1994). *Qualitative data analysis: An expanded sourcebook.* Thousand Oaks, CA: Sage.

Polit, D. F., & Beck, C. T. (2012). *Nursing research: Principles and methods* (9th ed.). Philadelphia, PA: Lippincott, Williams, & Wilkins.

Pope, C., Ziebland, S., & Mays, N. (2000). Analysing qualitative data. *British Medical Journal, 320*(7227), 114–116.

Van Manen, M. (1990). *Researching lived experience: Human science for an action sensitive pedagogy.* Albany, NY: State University of New York Press.

WRITING YOUR DISCUSSION CHAPTER

ELEMENTS OF YOUR DISCUSSION CHAPTER

1. A summary review of the problem

2. Key findings

3. What the findings mean in context of what is already known

4. Implications for practice, education, and policy

5. Future research

6. Limitations

7. Conclusion

This chapter covers how to write up your discussion. In this chapter, you'll learn how to write up a discussion of quantitative and qualitative results of a dissertation study and of a capstone project.

Here you are. You started out to make a meaningful contribution to nursing science and have spent years and untold effort on this work. Now you get to tell us all about it. The discussion chapter (Chapter Five) is your opportunity to lay out for your readers what your study means in the context of what is known or what is needed. And you explain how to take it and move forward to create changes or answer the next big question. The results you reported in the previous chapter (your results chapter, Chapter Four) are only raw material; the discussion is where you use that material to build something meaningful.

Begin this chapter as you have each of the others, with a brief description of what the chapter will cover.

A Review of the Problem

Begin with a brief review of what the problem is, a summary similar to what you did in the introduction, but much shorter. You need to remind readers of where it all began; they've probably read about 100 pages in between your introduction to the problem and this point. By reviewing some information here, you are reinforcing for the reader how what you discuss in this section relates to the purpose of your study or project.

Do not self-plagiarize from your introduction or literature review. You need to pull together the information from those chapters/sections and summarize them in one paragraph, two at the most.

Follow this summary with a restatement of your purpose statement, but now in the past tense. Then make a clear statement about what your key findings are and point out what contribution your study makes to the literature (what your study *adds*). The key findings should all relate to your research questions or the purpose of your project. The remaining findings, including those that were not statistically significant and incidental findings that are not directly related to your research questions, will be included in the discussion that follows, but they are not included here as a key finding.

EXAMPLE OF SUMMARY REVIEW AND KEY FINDINGS

This study, using both qualitative and quantitative methods, sought to understand the lived experience of women who experience IPV in a rural setting and the knowledge, attitudes, beliefs, and behaviors of healthcare providers.

The findings support and further illuminate results of the small body of research specific to IPV in a general population of women in a rural setting. Key findings include the self-imposed isolation that women engage in to manage stigma, the system-wide abuse by law enforcement and the legal system, and the resilience women demonstrate in overcoming multiple barriers to creating a new life separate from the abuser. Additionally, an encouraging key finding was the positive results of the healthcare provider survey, which found good knowledge, attitudes, beliefs, and behaviors related to IPV. Results of this study indicate that it is important that healthcare providers see their role in IPV as part of a broader integrated approach (Roush, 2014).

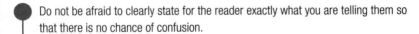

Do not be afraid to clearly state for the reader exactly what you are telling them so that there is no chance of confusion.

The key findings of this study are....

The contributions this study is making to the literature are....

Discussing Your Sample

Were there any interesting or surprising characteristics of your sample? For example, if a study in your topic area usually has a fairly even distribution between male and female participants and yours has a much higher percentage of men, you would point this out and refer to other studies to back up your claim that this is unusual, and then discuss possible reasons why it is different in your study.

Sample characteristics may also need to be discussed as you present your findings if you did subgroup analyses based on demographics. However, you should weave those into the discussion that follows.

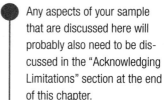

Any aspects of your sample that are discussed here will probably also need to be discussed in the "Acknowledging Limitations" section at the end of this chapter.

What Do Your Results Mean?

This is the heart of the discussion chapter. Here you tell your readers what the findings mean and put those findings in context of what is already known. Address each research question or variable that was in your study. Make sure that you discuss all the findings related to the questions or variables, including results that are not statistically significant. Point out surprising findings and talk about possible explanations for the results.

Avoid absolutisms. It is the rare study that can state anything categorically on its own. So don't use words like *unquestionably*, *undeniably*, *absolutely*, *definitely*, or *certainly* when talking about your findings. Also, be careful with use of terms such as *clearly shows* or *strongly indicates*. Do the strength of your findings (consider your study limitations here) support their use? Perhaps *suggests* or simply *indicates* without the qualifier would be a more accurate depiction of your findings.

EXAMPLE OF DISCUSSION OF SURPRISING FINDINGS

One of the most surprising findings of this investigation was the lack of correlation between levels of consistency with guidelines and clinical outcome. Several plausible explanations for this finding exist.

One factor that could have influenced these results was that there was less variability in the levels of consistency than anticipated. Fairly high levels of consistency between key elements of the CPTs and the interventions statements were found among all three intermediate clinical outcomes. The Principal Investigator anticipated that there would be some subjects who did not receive care that was consistent with guidelines; instead all subjects received care that was above the 50th percentile, making it harder to determine differences (Cunningham, 2003).

If you used a theoretical framework, discuss your results through the lens of the framework. There are a few different ways to accomplish this:

1. Focus a paragraph or two on how the results fit into the model.

2. Organize your discussion within the structure of the framework.

3. Integrate statements about how particular findings fit with the framework throughout the discussion.

EXAMPLE OF FOCUSING A PARAGRAPH ON HOW THE RESULTS FIT INTO THE MODEL

The findings clearly fall within Bronfenbrenner's ecological systems model, highlighting the need for a contextual approach to the problem of IPV in a rural setting. Acts of violence and patterns of abuse were made possible, and sustained, through cultural and societal archetypes at the macrosystem level. These archetypes—patriarchy, stigma, and discrimination—exerted a powerful influence on the women's lives through their impact on the exosystem and microsystem. At the exosystem level, they created financial hardship and difficulties with law enforcement and the legal system. At the microsystem level, they reinforced women's isolation from friends and family or colleagues, preventing them from developing a support system or social network of any kind. For some women, it meant the loss of their children. A lack of a social network constricted their opportunities to improve their economic situation and enabled problems with law enforcement and the legal system at the exosystem level. When caring for women who experience IPV, healthcare providers must consider elements of all these systems and be prepared to connect women with resources outside of the healthcare arena (Roush, 2014).

EXAMPLE OF INTEGRATION OF THEORETICAL FRAMEWORK IN DISCUSSION

In accordance with the relationship between concepts contained in Bandura's theory, there is a reciprocal relationship between strong self-efficacy beliefs and the accomplishment of determined behaviors or tasks whereby an increase in one enhances the other as well. People with high conviction in their capabilities sustain their efforts and are sure that they can exercise control (Bandura, 1982, 1997, 2000). Not only are self-efficacy beliefs and physical activity moderately positively correlated, but self-efficacy was the only variable that contributed to predicting physical activity. Nine percent of the variance in physical activity in the sample of Puerto Rican adults with type 2 DM can be explained by their self-efficacy beliefs (Davila, 2010).

Put your results in context of what we already know, and compare them to the results of previous studies. Do not just say that they were consistent or not consistent with previous studies; instead, give details. If the results are consistent with previous studies, provide examples of those studies, with details about the sample, method, and findings. Discuss how the congruency of results builds on or supports a particular hypothesis or existing practices or the current understanding of a phenomenon.

EXAMPLE OF CONSISTENT FINDINGS

One striking similarity between this study and Sellers et al. was that informants delay seeking out health care, especially during planting or harvest, and equate health with working or doing. Bushy (1997) has also identified that rural clients wait longer before they seek out health care. I found that in general these elders wait to go to the doctor until they can no longer do what they want to do and they define health as the ability to do. Pierce (2001), Weinert and Burman (1994), and Long and Weinert (1989) also identify that rural dwellers define health as the ability to do (Witt, 2006).

If the findings differ from previous findings, give examples as well, but also tell your readers how they differ and your thoughts about why they differ. What are the possible explanations for the difference? Was it related to different study populations or settings? Was it related to how a variable was measured or the instrument that was used? Does it have anything to do with changes in practice or policy since the earlier studies were done? Also discuss whether the differences bring into question existing practices or understanding of a phenomenon.

EXAMPLE OF EXPLANATION OF INCONSISTENT FINDINGS

There are several probable explanations for divergence in findings from multivariate analysis between this study and other studies available in the literature. First, control of confounders was either not present (Janssen et al., 2001; Shepley et al., 2008) or limited (Alimoglu & Donmez, 2005; Parish et al., 2008) in studies that found significant relationships between individual PWE features and job satisfaction, while the current study provided control of multiple confounders. Next, the current study used different PWE measures than measures used in other studies in which researchers either constructed their own measures (Janssen et al., 2001; Parish et al., 2008) or adapted existing measures without confirming validity and reliability of the adapted measure in the studied sample (Shepley et al., 2008) (Djukic, 2009).

You can refer readers back to a table or figure, or you can include data or details from your results when needed to enhance the discussion. For example, a quotation that wasn't included in the results chapter/section could be added to illustrate a point being made.

EXAMPLE OF DATA USED IN DISCUSSION

Women in this study did not have confidence in a protective order, viewing it as just "a piece of paper," a common perception among women who experience IPV. Women participating in a study of protective orders by Logan et al. (2005) also felt that the protective order was ineffective—viewing it as "just a piece of paper" (p. 891) as well. They reported that it was not enforced when there was a violation, a view also shared by women in this study. Women in Logan's study also cited fear of retaliation as a reason for not getting an order, a point of view noted very clearly by a woman in this study who said, "What are they going to do, slap them on the wrist and go yeah don't do it again? … Order of protection is just a piece of paper, and that's all it is, a piece of paper that sets people off more" (Roush, 2014).

Your discussion can expand into related areas to add context where appropriate. For example, in the example cited here (related to women not getting an order of protection, you could also bring in some of the research that looks at the effectiveness of protective orders, thus putting their decision in context of what we know.

EXAMPLE OF RELATED RESEARCH

Women's perceptions are supported by research that shows that the order of protection is generally ineffective in preventing future violence (McFarlane et al., 2004; Strand, 2012), except in cases where there was a low to moderate risk of repeated violence, though even then the effect was small. In the McFarlane et al. (2004) study, the researchers found that though there was no difference in subsequent violence against women who applied and got a restraining order and those who applied and did not get one; all of the women who applied experienced a lower level of violence in the following 18 months. They posited that the contact with the legal system may prevent future violence, but this is not consistent with the findings here, where most of the women had negative experiences with the legal system that further empowered the abuser. It may be characteristics of women who take the initiative to apply for a restraining order or the dynamics of their relationships that account for the differences (Roush, 2014).

As you talk about specific results, you can discuss ideas for possible solutions. Building on the protective order example, you can then go on to talk about strengthening the response of the legal system in enforcement of orders of protection to help change the perception women have about their effectiveness and thus increase their safety.

Discussing Implications for Practice, Education, Policy, and Research

Another important part of the discussion is telling your readers what the results mean out in the real world: the implications. What are your recommendations for applying the results to practice, education, policy, and research? You can talk about implications of each of the findings as you discuss them, or you can do it all together under a separate subsection. Either way, in most cases, you should address all four domains: practice, education, policy, and research. Not all of the findings will have implications for all four domains, but each of the four should be addressed at some point.

Practice

Do your findings raise questions about current standards of practice? Should current practice be changed based on your findings? If yes, how should it change? (Keep in mind, though, that it is rare that practice should be changed based on the results of just one study.) What specific actions should nurses take based on your findings? Do the findings reinforce current practice or changes to practice that have been proposed prior to your study?

Education

How do findings affect how nurses are being educated? Do they call for changes in the curriculum, and if yes, what changes? Do the findings suggest that a gap exists in nursing education? Do the findings indicate that current educational preparation related to your topic is not effective or that it is effective?

Policy

What policy changes need to happen based on your findings? What actions can nurses, at different levels or in varied settings, take to create needed policy changes?

Research

What is the next step in the research on this topic based on what your study has added to the knowledge? What do we need to know from here? Does this study need to be replicated with a larger sample or after addressing limitations you encountered? Does it need to be conducted in a different population or setting?

EXAMPLE OF RECOMMENDATION FOR RESEARCH

It was very difficult to recruit women for this study. It took 10 months to recruit the ultimate sample of 12 women needed to achieve saturation. Even then, all but two of the women had already left the abusive relationship. A challenge for future research is finding a way to include the most marginalized women in studies on IPV, including those who are still in the abusive relationship. Understanding their experiences is essential if we are to provide care and services that address the full spectrum of IPV experiences (Roush, 2014).

COMMON MISTAKE

Don't get carried away with implications and recommendations. Make sure that you can trace every implication and recommendation directly back to a finding in your study and that the finding is strong enough to support the recommendation.

You can organize your implications in a few different ways:

1. All together in their own subsection at the end of the discussion

2. Integrated into the discussion as you talk about each finding

3. A mix of the first two, with the domain (practice, education, research, policy) having the primary implications talked about as you go along and the others in a separate subsection at the end

For example, if you are doing a study or project that focuses on clinical care, it might flow better if you include the implications for *practice* for each finding as you talk about it, because the major implications are probably going to be those in the practice domain. Then, at the end of the discussion, you can include a subsection on implications for education, policy, and research.

> Write out your implications on a separate document before starting the discussion chapter/section. Make a table with five columns (see Table 5.1): Findings, Practice Implications, Education Implications, Policy Implications, and Research Implications. First list your findings in the first column. Then list all the possible implications and recommendations for each of the domains in the other columns.

In a capstone project, the implications include addressing sustainability of the quality improvement in your setting. Are you going to continue or expand on the project in your setting? As you move forward, how do you plan to address any of the challenges you encountered? If outcomes were not as anticipated or did not meet the goals, what are the plans for moving forward? In addition, you should discuss implications your project has outside of your immediate setting or with other patient populations.

Table 5.1   Table of Findings and Implications

Findings	Implications			
	Practice	*Education*	*Policy*	*Research*
Self-imposed Isolation	Public health outreach Universal screening	Educate Community Advocacy Survivors speak out		Recruit most marginalized Develop and test interventions to effectively improve healthcare providers' skills in identifying and managing IPV Use of Internet to reach and support marginalized women
System-wide abuse	Teams that include law enforcement, social workers, advocates, healthcare providers, and survivors Include information about legal resources on handouts given in clinical settings	Educate law enforcement Accountability Interprofessional education of law enforcement, healthcare providers, and others	Access to legal services Mandated health provider education National instead of state level policy regarding adjudication	Develop and test pre-qualification education programs Epidemiological studies of outcomes of IPV-related interactions with law enforcement and justice system
Resilience	Train survivors to lead support groups		Funding for services	Test programs that facilitate grassroots organization of survivors

Acknowledging Limitations

There is no such thing as a perfect study. Of course, you have done everything you could to ensure that you conducted a rigorous study, and you stand by your results. However, there will still be weaknesses. And that's okay as long as you take them into consideration and tell us what they are and what they mean for the results. Talk about the limitations in an objective tone. You are not making excuses for them; instead, you are just stating what they are and what effect they may have on the results. If you took any actions to mitigate the effect, state those as well.

The following subsections describe some of the more common limitations that come up in studies.

Bias

Discuss anything that may have introduced or allowed for bias in your results. This might be related to your sample (for example, convenience sample), setting (one local urban clinic and, therefore, may not be representative of other settings), recruitment strategy (email, so only reached those who use email), or final sample (high or low percentage of certain demographic characteristic). It can also be related to your method of data collection (computer-based, for example, so only those with computers could participate; or people were asked to remember something, and so there may be recall bias).

Generalizability

Can your findings be generalized outside of the sample group and setting? If not, why not? This would not apply to qualitative research, but you should still address it and make a statement that generalizability is not sought in qualitative research and cite an expert-authored text to support that.

Reliability and Validity

Was there anything about the data collection that may have affected the reliability or validity of your results? Were the instruments used tested in your sampling population? Was inter-rater reliability a consideration?

EXAMPLES OF REPORT OF LIMITATIONS

There was the risk of response bias, since the sample are women who volunteered to participate and they may differ from those who would not volunteer: They recognize that their experiences constituted IPV and they had the resources to respond. Also, the women who have the resources and ability (such as transportation) to participate may not represent the more marginalized population of abused women, nor does it represent women who experience IPV yet do not label it as such (Roush, 2014).

Another limitation is that patients in the datasets can be represented more than one time. The unit of analysis for developing and evaluating the indices was episode of care defined as a maximum of 60 days. This could bias results as patient health characteristics could be correlated from one episode to another (Heckman, 1990).

However, as previously mentioned, 67% of the patients were on their first episode. Furthermore, there was only an average 1.5 episodes per patient. Therefore, correlated episodes are unlikely to bias the results found in this dissertation (Scharpf, 2005).

Crafting Your Conclusion

This is it: the final word. Way back when you started out with a germ of an idea related to something you felt strongly about. You made us care about it, too. You designed a study, collected and analyzed data, and interpreted the results. What are the major points you want readers to take away from this work? This is your final opportunity to drill it home.

You may want to begin your conclusion with a clear restatement of the major finding of your study or the major implication of your capstone project before going to the take-home message.

> *This study indicates that post-discharge follow-up care by a nurse practitioner can improve outcomes for heart failure patients and reduce readmissions.*

> *The outcomes of this project reinforce the importance of involving all members of the healthcare team in transitional care communication strategies.*

The conclusion should not be much more than a few paragraphs. Be concise and clear. Don't be afraid to make strong statements based on the evidence you've generated. Remember, you're an expert now.

COMMON MISTAKE

Don't just restate your key findings and summary from the discussion. That's all been said already. Pull it all together and take it up a notch. Imagine you are telling someone about your study or project and they looked at you somewhat skeptically and asked, "So what?" Then write your answer.

EXAMPLE OF CONCLUSION

Intimate partner violence is a public health problem that requires a coordinated interprofessional approach to prevention and management. The results of this study illustrate the complex web of individual, social, cultural, economic, and political factors that create and feed the problem. Many of the issues raised by the participants, such as discrimination, social isolation, financial constraints, and problems with the legal system, originate outside of the healthcare system. Therefore, the solution must go beyond one-on-one interactions between victims and their healthcare providers, no matter how knowledgeable and well intentioned the provider may be. Healthcare providers must provide care within a network of social workers, law-enforcement personnel, judiciary officials, counselors, and advocates. Ideally, whoever a victim first engages with should be able to facilitate connections with resources anywhere within such a network.

Finally, until we address the sociocultural factors of oppression and patriarchy that underlie much of the discrimination and disparities encountered by the women in this study, intimate partner violence will continue to be a devastating health and social problem for so many women. Advocacy and policy development must be undertaken as part of a comprehensive public-health approach (Roush, 2014).

That's it. You're done with the write-up. Next step—your oral defense. Nerve-wracking yes, but you are ready, and you'll do great. You'll walk into that room a doctoral candidate, an ABD. And you'll walk out as one of a very select group, currently less than 1% of nurses, as a matter of fact…

You'll walk out of there as a doctor.

Good luck and congratulations!

Chapter Checkup

❏ Have I provided a brief review of the problem?

❏ Have I highlighted the key findings?

❏ Have I noted any unusual characteristics in the sample population?

❏ Have I discussed how the findings fit into the theoretical model?

❏ Have I discussed how my findings are similar to or different from those of previous studies and provided possible explanations for those differences?

❏ Is everything I discuss directly related to the purpose statement, or does it provide context that enhances the reader's understanding of the findings?

❏ Have I included implications for practice, education, policy, and research?

❏ Are recommendations consistent with the findings?

❏ Have I addressed how I plan on sustaining practice or process changes for a quality-improvement project?

❏ Have I addressed unanticipated outcomes of a quality-improvement project?

❏ Have I included plans for addressing challenges encountered during implementation of a quality-improvement project?

❏ Have I described the study limitations?

❏ Is my conclusion consistent with and supported by the findings?

References

Cunningham, R. S. (2003). *Advanced practice nursing interventions and outcomes: An exploration of transitional care services post prostatectomy* (Doctoral dissertation, University of Pennsylvania). Available from ProQuest Dissertations and Theses database. (305307337)

Davila, N. (2010). *Physical activity in Puerto Rican adults with type 2 diabetes mellitus* (Doctoral dissertation). Retrieved from http://arizona.openrepository.com/ arizona/handle/10150/195609

Djukic, M. (2009). *Physical work environment: Testing an expanded job satisfaction model in a sample of hospital staff registered nurses* (Doctoral dissertation, New York University). Available from ProQuest Dissertations and Theses database. (3382425)

Roush, K. (2014). *The experience of intimate partner violence in the context of the rural setting* (Doctoral dissertation, New York University). Available from ProQuest Dissertations and Theses database. (1551746532)

Scharpf, T. P. (2005). *Functional status and quality in home health care* (Doctoral dissertation, Case Western Reserve University). Available from ProQuest Dissertations and Theses database. Retrieved from http://search.proquest.com/docview/305006 546?accountid=27880 (305006546)

Witt, D. E. (2006). *Growing old on the farm: An ethnonursing examination of aging and health within the agrarian rural subculture* (Doctoral dissertation, Duquesne University). Available from ProQuest Dissertations and Theses database.

Resources

Polit, D. F., & Beck, C. T. (2012). *Nursing research: Principles and methods* (9th ed.). Philadelphia, PA: Lippincott, Williams, & Wilkins.

Polkinghorne, D.E. (2007). Validity issues in narrative research. *Qualitative Inquiry, 13*(4), 471–486.

6

WRITING WELL:
THE BASICS

Contrary to popular belief, scholarly papers don't have to be
dull and tedious. You're writing about something you think is
important. So you want to communicate that importance. The way
to do that is through writing that has energy and voice, *your* voice.
In the process of doing a dissertation or capstone project, you will
become an expert in your topic; you've read all the literature and
been out in the field. So, write with a strong voice. Be direct and
confident.

Good scholarly writing engages readers and holds their attention from the first sentence to the last. It doesn't leave the slightest room for misinterpretation. You accomplish that by using language that is clear, engaging, and straightforward and by organizing the paper so that your readers are carried along smoothly through the material. Along with these elements that are essential to all writing, scholarly writing requires that you are accurate and avoid bias.

Four key characteristics are present in all good writing, and you need to strive for these in yours: clarity, conciseness, specificity, and good organization.

Achieving Clarity

Clarity ensures that what you write will be understood the way you mean it to be by *everyone* who reads your paper. Clear writing doesn't leave room for confusion or error. You can ensure clarity in a number of ways. One of the most important is your use of language. Along with language is the importance of correct grammar, particularly sentence structure. Being concise and specific will also enhance clarity, as you will see as they are discussed later in this chapter.

Choosing Your Language

There is a saying among writers that you should never use a $100 word when a $5 word will do. This is a particular problem in academic writing, where we are trying to communicate complex information and often think we need to use big, important words to do it. When actually, simple, everyday language is always best. Straightforward language is more concise and specific. I'm not talking about "dumbing down" information or not using technical or medical terms where needed. It's about writing *use* instead of *utilize* or *agree* instead of *are in agreement.*

Here's another example:

Overly complex and awkward: *The participant maintained eyelid closure for 5 minutes.*

Simple and clear: *The participant closed her eyes for 5 minutes.*

As you write, keep in mind that your goal is to communicate clearly, not to impress readers with your vocabulary.

You'll find a list of $100 words and phrases and their alternates at the end of the chapter.

Use the Active Voice

The active voice injects energy into your writing. In the active voice, the subject acts upon the object. In contrast, in the passive voice, the subject is being acted upon:

- **Passive:** The medication was injected by the nurse.
- **Active:** The nurse injected the medication.

The active voice is strong, direct, and concise. The passive voice lacks energy, is wordier, and can obscure meaning. However, in a couple of situations, you might want to use a passive voice: if the subject (doer) is unknown or unimportant, or if you want to emphasize the action or object rather than the subject.

For example, in a paper on medication errors, a sentence talking about an incident involving a child is written in passive voice in order to emphasize that this was a child whose life was endangered, rather than emphasize who made the error.

> *The 3-year-old child was given an adult dose of the medication....*

When you do a spell and grammar check, it will usually indicate which sentences are in passive voice and make suggestions for rewriting them in active voice. Do not automatically follow spell-check recommendations; make sure they work for your sentence. It will also give you an overall percentage of sentences that are in passive voice. You want to aim for as close to zero as you can get, but definitely keep it under 10%. If it comes out higher, read through the document and look for sentences that contain any version of *be* (*is*, *was*, *were*, *am*, *are*, or *been*) or that contain the word *by*.

Use I (It's Okay!)

A myth in academic writing holds that it is not scholarly to use personal pronouns. When you read some research reports, it's as if no humans were involved in conducting studies or analyzing results. Avoiding the use of personal pronouns leads to all kinds of bad writing: passive voice, less clarity, anthropomorphization, and lots of extra words. Take a look at the following to see the difference:

> *A project was conducted by the author to determine whether ....*

> *I conducted a study to determine whether ....*

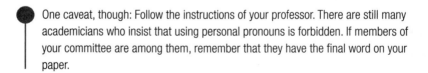

One caveat, though: Follow the instructions of your professor. There are still many academicians who insist that using personal pronouns is forbidden. If members of your committee are among them, remember that they have the final word on your paper.

AVOIDING ANTHROPOMORPHIZATION

Anthropomorphization is giving human characteristics to nonhuman entities. Here are a couple of examples of how it can manifest in a dissertation or capstone project report.

Incorrect: This research found a correlation between nurse fatigue and medication error rates.

Correct: The researchers found a correlation between nurse fatigue and medication error rates.

Incorrect: This project will attempt to increase medication adherence through the use of telephone follow-up post-discharge.

Correct: I will attempt to increase medication adherence through the use of telephone follow-up post-discharge.

or

The purpose of this project is to increase medication adherence through the use of telephone follow-up post-discharge.

Check Your Adjectives at the Door

When it comes to adjectives, the fewer the better. You rarely need more than one, at most two, descriptors. And avoid intensifiers, words such as *somewhat, quite,* and *very.* Not only are they inexact and subjective, they also imply uncertainty or a reluctance to commit to a statement.

Do not to slip into hyperbole. Words such as *distraught, catastrophic, devastating,* or *agony* lose meaning and power unless used sparingly and appropriately. There are health problems that are devastating, and patients' pain may reach the level of agony, but you will lose credibility if you overstate descriptions of situations.

Go through your paper and remove all the adjectives and intensifiers. Now read the paper. Put back in only those that are absolutely needed.

Be Concrete

Avoid abstract nouns. Abstract nouns represent things that are intangible; you can't see, hear, touch, smell, or taste them. Abstract nouns are subjective; they are interpreted through the lens of each reader's own experiences, and the meaning they give to it may differ from what you intended. Concrete nouns represent something tangible; you can see, hear, touch, smell, or taste it. When you use concrete nouns, you control the image created in the reader's mind. See Table 6.1 for some examples.

Table 6.1 Examples of Concrete and Abstract Nouns

Concrete Nouns	Abstract Nouns
Women	Childhood
Man	Health
Nurse	Caring
Stretcher	Patience
Building	Energy
Juice	Independence
Suture	Kindness
Clock	Love

Avoid Jargon

Jargon is specialized vocabulary used by members of a group. Nursing has a lot of jargon (such as *call a code*, *draw blood*, *run fluids*, and *stat*), and for most of us it has become such an ingrained part of our vocabulary that we don't even realize it is jargon anymore. There are a couple of problems with jargon:

- It is exclusionary; people outside of the group don't understand it.

- It leaves room for misinterpretation.

Some healthcare jargon can be so specialized that people outside of a region or particular healthcare setting may misinterpret it. When I worked in upstate New York, we referred to a cardiac arrest in the hospital I worked in as a *Dr. Core* because that was how it was called over the hospital-wide intercom system. I never realized that it was a local expression until I moved away and started working at another hospital, where a cardiac arrest was called a *Code Blue* and no one had ever heard the term *Dr. Core*.

Also avoid the use of euphemisms. Euphemisms are terms we use in place of words or phrases that communicate something that is difficult to talk about. For example, one of the most common euphemisms is the term *passed away* in place of *died*.

Checking Your Grammar

Numerous good resources are available, both online and in print, for checking punctuation and grammar. *Use them.* This section examines a couple of areas where new writers often make errors that can result in confusion and misunderstanding for the reader: differentiating between the use of colons, semicolons, and commas and using *misplaced modifiers* and *dangling participles*.

Punctuation

Punctuation clarifies meaning in a sentence, guides the reader through the material, and alerts the reader to where the emphasis is. Punctuation is straightforward for the most part, but three punctuation marks that are used frequently and often incorrectly are commas, colons, and semicolons.

The *colon* has a simple purpose: introduction. Most often it is used to introduce a list of things—Marla gathered all the supplies for the dressing change: sterile gloves, sterile saline, gauze pads, an ace wrap, and tape. But, it can also be used to introduce a single thing, adding emphasis (as in the first sentence of this paragraph). However, you should not use a colon after a verb—Marla gathered: sterile gloves, sterile saline, gauze pads, rolled gauze, and tape.

The *semicolon* gets a little more complicated because its usage is often confused with that of the comma. The semicolon is used when two related sentences are connected in a single sentence without using a conjunction; a comma is used when two sentences are connected with a conjunction. The semicolon is also used when a sentence lists multiple complex items that have commas. It tells the reader what goes together—Marla gathered what she needed for the dressing change, including sterile gloves, saline, and gauze pads; an ace wrap and tape; and a disposal bag for the old dressing.

The *comma* is the most complicated of all because it has many uses. It is used to separate items in a series, separate two complete sentences with the use of a conjunction, separate a nonessential phrase in the middle of a sentence, and to attach words to the beginning or end of a sentence.

Misplaced Modifiers and Dangling Participles

A modifier is a word or phrase that modifies a noun or verb. A participle is a particular type of modifier, usually ending in –*ing*. The modifier should be as close as possible to what it is modifying. When it's not, that's when you get into trouble.

Take a look at the following sentence and think about what it is actually saying.

> *Simulation is used in various nursing and medical specialties including critical care and surgery to enhance clinical judgment, critical thinking, and communication.*

The modifier is "to enhance clinical judgment, critical thinking, and communication." The closest thing to it is "surgery," so that is what it is modifying. According to this sentence, there is surgery that will enhance clinical judgment, critical thinking, and communication!

Here is the sentence corrected so that the modifier is closest to what it is actually modifying, "simulation."

> *Simulation is used to enhance clinical judgment, critical thinking, and communication in various nursing and medical specialties, including critical care and surgery.*

It's hard to catch your own misplaced modifiers. You know what you are trying to say, so you read what you've written as saying what you intended it to say instead of reading what it actually says. This is one of the reasons it's so important to get others to read your drafts and give you feedback.

Being Concise

Concise writing is accurate, clear, and engaging. You don't want any extraneous words and phrases; every word in your paper should be doing a job. Don't leave it up to the reader to try to separate the superfluous from the important; that is your job. If a lot of "stuff" clutters your message, the message loses impact and may get lost completely.

Use of straightforward language and an active voice are key to concise writing. You also need to be on the lookout for redundancy. Often we repeat information or say the same thing in different ways when we are trying to ensure we are being clear. In actuality, though, repetition is more likely to muddy the picture. If you use specific details and straightforward language, you will be clear and need only say something once.

In addition, we use many redundant expressions in our speech and writing. Consider, for example, the following statement:

> *There was general consensus among the committee members that staffing needed to be increased during the night shift.*

Consensus means *general agreement*. So, when you write that there was general consensus, you are saying that there was general general agreement. You can simply say there was consensus.

A list of commonly used redundant phrases and terms is included at the end of the chapter.

Being Specific

Generalities leave a lot of room for misinterpretation or misdirection. You may begin a section or paragraph with a general statement, but you then need to drill down into specific details. Scientific writing needs to be precise. Studies need to be reported with a level of detail that will allow others to replicate them; the same is true of quality-improvement projects. The use of concrete nouns, as described earlier in this chapter, is essential for specificity.

Lacking specificity: Members of the committee held training sessions to introduce the new policy. The sessions took place over 2 weeks and were available for all the nurses. The committee members focused training on the parts of the new policy that nurses needed, either the new parts or the entire procedure, and made sure all the nurses knew the evidence behind it. They also posted information on the units.

Version with specificity: Members of the committee held 1-hour training sessions over 2 weeks to introduce the new policy. They scheduled the sessions at varied times so that nurses on all shifts were able to attend. If nurses were familiar with the new policy, we focused on the changes. If nurses were not familiar with the new policy, we reviewed the entire policy and highlighted the changes. All the training sessions included an overview of the evidence used to develop the policy. In addition to training sessions, information sheets were posted in each of the nursing stations next to the medication cart.

Being Organized

When your paper is well organized, the reader will move through the paper smoothly: no bumps, disruptions, or surprises. Each idea, sentence, paragraph, and section logically connects to what came before and what follows.

- Ideas should flow from general to specific.

- Make sure that no ideas or statements come out of nowhere; introduce an idea or concept before you discuss it. Double-check this whenever you move things around during revisions.

- If you state you're going to cover a, b, and c, then discuss a, then b, and then c. Don't talk about b, then a, and then c.

- There should be only *one* main idea to a paragraph.

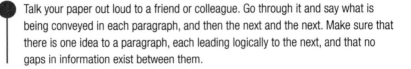

Talk your paper out loud to a friend or colleague. Go through it and say what is being conveyed in each paragraph, and then the next and the next. Make sure that there is one idea to a paragraph, each leading logically to the next, and that no gaps in information exist between them.

Making Clear Transitions

When a manuscript is well organized, readers are prepared for changes in ideas or focus as they move through the paper. This is accomplished with the use of transitional devices: words and phrases that connect ideas, paragraphs, and sections. Transitional devices do more than just connect these elements; they also indicate relationships between them. They guide the reader in how to think about the relationships. For example, *however* tells the reader, "Wait a minute, there's also *this*, which makes us think a little differently about *that*."

Be careful with transitional devices. Don't just pop in the first one that comes to mind or use the same one over and over. A common mistake is the use of transitions that indicate relationships where none exist or are not what the transitional word or phrase indicates. The use of *therefore* is a common example of this; it indicates that because of *that*, we can now think or do *this*. Make sure that such a relationship really exists.

Transitional words and phrases are also used when there is a shift in focus between paragraphs and sections. They summarize what was just said, prepare the reader for what comes next, and make a connection between them. They say, "Pay attention here, we were talking about *that*, but now we are going to talk about *this*, which is *connected* in this way." Notice how the first sentence of the second paragraph in the following excerpt does this:

> *Obstetric fistula is an outcome of obstructed labor; labor that will sometimes go on for days. The prolonged pressure of the infant's skull against the soft tissue of the birth canal leads to ischemia and necrosis of the surrounding tissue, leaving a hole between the vagina and bladder (vesico-vaginal) or sometimes between the rectum and bladder (recto-vaginal), or both. The woman is left with constant leakage of urine or feces and develops an offensive odor, sores on her perineum and upper legs, and infections. Most of the women are also grieving the loss of their baby; studies report infant mortality rates from 85% to 100% in cases of childbirth that result in an obstetric fistula.* [1], [3] and [4]

> *The worst suffering for these women though may not be the physical manifestations of obstetric fistula or grief over the loss of their baby, but rather the social repercussions that follow. The majority of women who suffer an obstetric fistula already live in precarious socioeconomic circumstances compli-cated by the low status of women in sub-Saharan Africa; they are usually poor, uneducated, from a rural area of subsistence farmers, and unskilled.* [1] *Many are really only girls, as young as 14 or 15, married off shortly after puberty with a first pregnancy following soon after* [1] and [5] *(Roush, 2009, p. e21).*

The first paragraph is talking about the physical consequences of obstetric fistula, including infant death. The second paragraph begins with a sentence that tells us what we just read; prepares us that there are other, perhaps worse, things to consider; and then goes on to say what those are.

Revise, Revise, Revise

Leave yourself plenty of time for multiple revisions. When you finish a draft of a chapter, set it aside for a few days. Then come back to it and read it out loud. Reading aloud requires more attention and gives you a sense of the flow. You will hear or feel the places where it isn't working: the gaps you fall into, the places where you get lost in endless sentences, the bumpy connections. Then revise and do the same thing again. When your entire dissertation or capstone is finished, read it out loud again (yes, the *entire* thing).

You should also get two other people to read your work and give you feedback. One should be a person who knows the topic well and who can give you feedback on accuracy and point out gaps in information. The other should be someone who knows nothing about the topic (in fact, preferably someone outside of nursing or healthcare). If your second reader can follow and understand it, you know your writing is clear and complete.

The Chapter Checkup on pp. 124–125 of this chapter is a handy revision checklist you can use to help your revision process.

Double-check that all the references you list in your reference list are in the final paper and vice versa. It's easy for some to get missed, either left out or not deleted when they should be, when you do multiple revisions. Print out your reference list. Use the Find Command (Ctrl+F) to look through your paper for each reference on the list, and check it off when you find it. Then go back through the paper and check that each reference cited in the paper is on the reference list.

Following is a list of writing tips based on errors often seen in dissertations and capstone project:

- *Data* is plural. *Datum* is singular.

- Et al. has a period only after the al.

- Only capitalize proper nouns. This might seem like an easy one, but a lot of people get it wrong. When talking about a theory, you capitalize only the name of the person involved, not each word of the theory. So, you would write Bronfenbrenner's ecological systems model, not Bronfenbrenner's Ecological Systems Model. The same is true of conditions and diseases. You don't write Alzheimer's Disease or Cognitive Behavioral Therapy. You do write Alzheimer's disease and cognitive behavioral therapy.

- Go through your final paper carefully to make sure that all the tenses in each chapter are correct. See the guidelines in Chapter 2, "Writing Your Literature Review," for guidance. It is easy to miss a few in a paper of 100 or 200 pages when you are going back to change them after you have completed your study.

- Check your *it's* and *its*. *It's* is a contraction of it is. *Its* is a possessive.

- Use the same term for a concept or variable throughout the paper. You can even keep a list of such key concepts or variables to ensure you use them consistently throughout.

- Avoid long, overly complex sentences. The reader can get lost or confused wading through them.

- Avoid labels. They introduce bias. For example, instead of "disabled patients," write "patients with disabilities."

$100 Words and Phrases

a large majority of = most

are in agreement = agree

at this point in time = now

attempt, endeavor = try

be in the possession of = possess, own

be of the opinion = think, believe, feel

by means of = by

commence = begin

due to the fact that, owing to the fact, in light of the fact, in view of the fact = because

facilitate = help, assist, ease

for the purpose of = for, to

has the capacity of = can

implement = do, perform, carry out

in the event that = if

incentivize = motivate, stimulate, spur

individual = person, woman, man (unless you are distinguishing a person from a group)

on a daily basis or *on a regular basis* = daily or regularly *optimize/maximize* = increase, improve, expand

possess = have

prior to, previous to, in advance of = before

subsequent to = after, following

take into consideration = consider

utilization = use (noun)

utilize = use (verb)

with the exception of = except

Redundancies

A new initiative

Absolutely necessary

Artificial prosthesis

Each and every

General consensus

Interact with each other

Interact with one another

Just recently

Repeat again

Self-confessed

Sufficient enough

The reason is because

Chapter Checkup

❏ Organization

   Do ideas flow from general to specific?

   Do ideas follow through from the beginning?

   Do any ideas/statements come out of nowhere?

   Is there redundancy?

   Is there one main idea in each paragraph?

❏ Transitions

   Are there transitional statements between ideas?

   Are there transitional statements between paragraphs and sections?

❏ Is tense consistent throughout?

❏ Language

   Is language straightforward?

   Have I used simple terms rather than pretentious, showy words?

   Is the language free of jargon?

   Is the language concise?

   Are the nouns I use concrete and specific?

   Have I avoided using hyperbole and multiple descriptors?

   Are all adjectives and adverbs absolutely necessary?

   Have I used the same term for a concept throughout?

❏ Have I used primarily the active voice?

❏ Grammar

 Is there parallel construction?

 Have I checked for misplaced modifiers and dangling participles?

 Does punctuation use meet accepted standards?

 Is it clear who or what each pronoun is referring to?

❏ Synthesis

 Have I synthesized information vs. listing information?

❏ Have I gotten feedback?

Remember: CLARITY IS KEY.

The Scholar's Voice© 2009

References

Roush, K. (2009). Social implications of obstetric fistula in women in sub-Saharan Africa: An integrative review. *Journal of Midwifery and Women's Health*, *54*(2), e21-e33.

INDEX

F

G

H–I

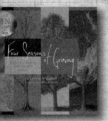
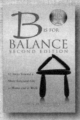
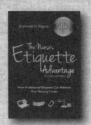
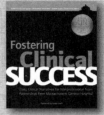
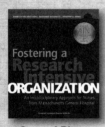
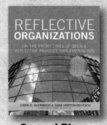
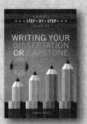

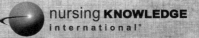

Tools for Researchers

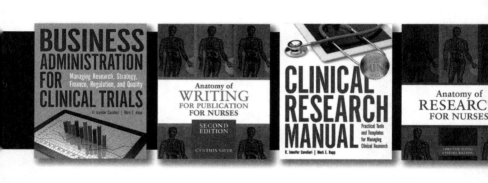

Business Administration for Clinical Trials

By R. Jennifer Cavalieri and Mark E. Rupp

Anatomy of Writing for Publication for Nurses, Second Edition

By Cynthia Saver

Clinical Research Manual

By R. Jennifer Cavalieri and Mark E. Rupp

Anatomy of Research for Nurses

By Christine Hedges Barbara Williams

To order, visit **www.nursingknowledge.org/sttibooks**.
Discounts are available for institutional purchases.
Call **888.NKI.4YOU** for details.

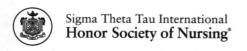

Sigma Theta Tau International
Honor Society of Nursing®

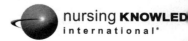

nursing **KNOWLED**
i n t e r n a t i o n a l®